SOLO's Field Guide to
Wilderness
First Aid
Afloat

Wilderness and Marine Medicine

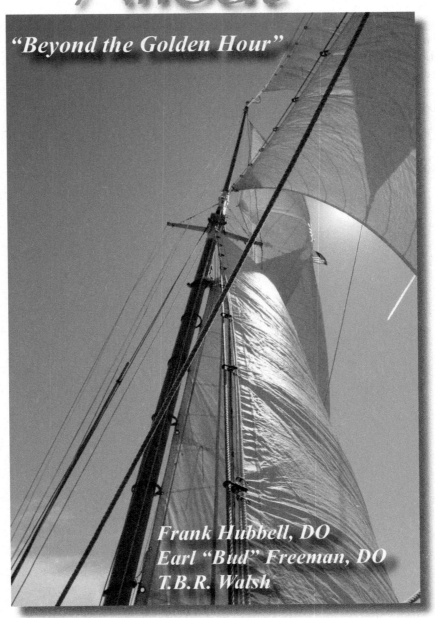

"Beyond the Golden Hour"

Frank Hubbell, DO
Earl "Bud" Freeman, DO
T.B.R. Walsh

SOLO'S FIELD GUIDE TO WILDERNESS FIRST AID AFLOAT

Published by:
TMC Books/Stonehearth Open Learning Opportunities
731 Tasker Hill Rd., Conway, NH 03818
info@TMCBooks.com
http://www.TMCbooks.com
http://www.soloschools.com

ISBN: 978-0-9826539-2-0

TMC books LLC

731 Tasker Hill Road
Conway, NH 03818
www.tmcbooks.com

This book is dedicated
to Saxon, our canine companion and
veteran sailor. She has made many a
voyage.
And to all the Good Samaritans who
have the heart to stop and help.

Jesus replied and said, "A certain man was going down from Jerusalem to Jericho; and he fell among robbers, and they stripped him and beat him , and went off leaving him half dead.

"And by chance a certain priest was going down on that road, and when he saw him, he passed by on the other side.

"And likewise a Levite also, when he came to the place and saw him, passed by on the other side.

"But a certain Samaritan, who was on a journey, came upon him; and when he saw him, he felt compassion, and came to him, and bandaged up his wounds, pouring oil and wine on them; and he put him on his own beast, and brought him to an inn, and took care of him."

Luke 10:30-34
NAS

SOLO's Field Guide to Wilderness First Aid Afloat

The SOLO Field Guide to Wilderness First Aid Afloat is the manual that accompanies SOLO's two-day course of the same name. The Wilderness First Aid Afloat (WFA Afloat) course was created out of the direct experience of the founders of SOLO and is designed by and for the "outdoor enthusiast:" whether kayaker, canoeist, sailor, or power boater, who spends recreation time on the water. It is for the adventurous who may find themselves away from immediate help and may have to rely on their own skills to survive and thrive if an emergency should arise.

First offered in 1974 under the name of the Mountain Rescue Seminar, the course next became Backcountry Medicine, and eventually Wilderness First Aid, and in this version, has been adapted for water entusiasts. The course has continued to evolve over the past 33 years, through over a thousand programs, and more than 50,000 students.

A jam-packed, fast-paced course, WFA Afloat covers a variety of topics including how to recognize and manage common medical problems along with rare but life-threatening emergencies, environmental emergencies, and most importantly, prevention of these problems. This textbook is intended to be a true field guide that our students can carry with them throughout their training with SOLO and use as a reference later.

The curriculum of the SOLO Field Guide to Wilderness First Aid Afloat has been approved by the United States Coast Guard

This is a course in First Aid and prevention. It is not a boater safety course, a water rescue course, or a white-water rescue course, and is not meant to take the place of, or subsitute for, those courses.

SOLO enthusiastically recommends additional safety training as part of accident prevention on the water.

Table of Contents

Editor's Note: *We extend our apologies to grammarians for the often unorthodox use of punctuation marks and capital letters and for the intentional lack of agreement between pronouns and their antecedents.*

THE "MARINE" IN WILDERNESS FIRST AID AFLOAT:

WHAT IS "WILDERNESS AND MARINE" AND WHY IS IT SO CHALLENGING TO THE EMERGENCY CAREGIVER?

In the world of pre-hospital medicine, the term "wilderness" or "extended care" is defined as any time a patient is more than an hour from definitive (hospital ER) care. The critical first hour after an injury occurs is called the "Golden Hour."

In the wilderness or marine setting it is very easy to consume hours in a rescue effort. When someone becomes sick or injured, a chain of events has to occur to get the patient off of the high seas and into the hospital, and it is more than simply calling 911. Commonly, someone has to radio out and notify EMS or the Coast Guard; then those called have to respond to the scene and to locate the patient, treat and package the patient, transfer them out to the waiting ambulance, and finally transport them to the hospital.

Time, Distance, and Response: it's farther and longer than you think.

- Rapid notification for help is maybe impossible.
- Informtion may have to be relayed by radio or cell phone.
- The response by the rescue team may be prolonged. What will you do until help arrives?
- Provision of emergency care is clearly outside the "Golden Hour."

Even though most boaters might be able to radio, or call the outside world,

amost all boating accidents happen outside the "Golden Hour".

The Environment: if not already hostile, it can easily turn hostile.

- Cold, wet, wind, driving snow, high seas, and even darkness can delay rescuers even longer.
- Poor weather conditions can be a direct threat to the safety of rescuers, the patient, and others with the patient.
- Poor weather conditions may eliminate the possibility of access by helicopter.
- It can be much more difficult to take care of yourself, the patient, and anyone else on the scene.

Think about the enviornment: it can be hazardous and make movement slow.

- Access to the patient might require special skills due to high seas or the size of the vessel.

- Stabilizing the patient may be extremely difficult on a moving deck.

- The patient may be diificult to reach due to confined space aboard; or in the case of paddlers, they might not even be in the same boat.

Equipment and Resources: maximize efficiency to minimize weight.

- Is the group to be rescued prepared for the conditions?
- Is the responding team "wilderness" trained and prepared for the conditions?
- The group must know how to improvise equipment.
- Limited equipment and access to resources is the norm.

> The U.S. Coast Guard requires certain safety equipment be on board and accessible on all recreational vessels for very good reasons. The number of required items varies with the size and type of vessel; however, the USCG requirements are the minimums and do not include luxury items like anchors, tow lines, food, fresh water, or warm clothing.

Specialized Training and Wilderness Knowledge: get smart.

- Navigation, understanding of tides and currents.
- Weather forecasting skills.
- Basic water safety training.
- Technical rescue skills, ropes and knots, water rescue skills.
- Understanding long-term patient care.
- Helicopter rescue training.

For all of these reasons wilderness/marine care providers are expected to follow and to perform at a different standard of care than a care provider in an urban setting. As implied, someone learning wilderness or marine first aid may need to learn and master a number of skills that are not directly related to patient care. They may also be expected to manage an injury differently than a caregiver in an urban environment simply because the remote care provider may be staying with the patient for a long time while waiting for help to arrive, and possibly while the patient is being transported to definitive care.

— *NOTES* —

CHAPTER ONE

RESPONSE AND ASSESSMENT

What happened?

BODY SUBSTANCE ISOLATION (BSI):
Also referred to as Total Fluid Precautions or Universal Precautions

In providing emergency medical care you can be exposed to infectious disease agents, and you need to know how to protect yourself against these disease-causing organisms.

Modes of Transmission

DIRECT CONTACT

The spread of disease by direct contact with the blood or other body substances of an infected individual (saliva, sputum, blood, urine, feces, secretions).

INDIRECT CONTACT

The spread of disease from one individual to another by touching a contaminated inanimate object (door knob, clothing, stretcher, countertop, etc.) and then transferring the pathogen to mouth or eyes with the now contaminated hands.

AIRBORNE

The spread of disease by infected droplets of saliva or sputum expelled into the air by coughing or sneezing and then being inhaled by another person.

VECTOR

The spread of disease by blood-sucking insects, such as mosquitoes, fleas, or ticks.

WATERBORNE

The spread of disease by the consumption of contaminated water, usually contaminated with human waste, the "oral fecal route."

Our primary defense is behavior: we take precautions to prevent contamination.
PREVENTION equals BEHAVIOR.

GLOVES OR WATERPROOF BARRIER

To prevent DIRECT CONTACT, establish a barrier before any potential exposure to body fluids.

HAND-WASHING

To prevent patient-to-patient and hand-to-mouth transfer of pathogens by INDIRECT CONTACT, wash hands before and after any patient contact.

MASKS

To prevent AIRBORNE spread, put on a surgical mask before any potential exposure to airborne pathogens, especially tuberculosis (put a mask on the patient, too, if possible).

INSECT REPELLENT, MOSQUITO NETTING, CLOTHING

To prevent the transmission of disease by blood-sucking insects, use insect repellents (Permethrin), wear protective clothing, sleep under mosquito netting, and do tick checks.

WATER PURIFICATION

To prevent waterborne illnesses always make and drink potable water by boiling, use of water filters, chemicals (iodine or chlorine), or the use of UVC light (Steripen).

THE ANATOMY OF A CRISIS: THE PATIENT ASSESSMENT SYSTEM

What would you do if you were out in your boat and were the first one to arrive at the scene of an accident?

- How would you find out what is wrong and what has happened?
- How do you tell how badly hurt the injured person is?
- Do you go for help?
- Do you try to help the injured person?
- What should you do?

The method used is STOP and Survey referred to as *The Patient Assessment System* which consists of a list of questions and tasks that need to be performed in order to ascertain what happened and what you are going to do about it.

- These questions and tasks are arranged by priority and should be done in order.
- You should not move on to the next task until the one you are on has been successfully completed.

Part 1—STOP—SCENE SURVEY: Is the scene safe?

- Are you safe? Seamanship remains a priority–wind, current, sea conditions–securing the safety of the boat is of prime importance to everyone on board.
- Is everyone else safe?
- Is the patient safe?
- What happened? (Mechanism of Injury—MOI)
- How do you safely approach the victim?
- What is your general impression of the situation's seriousness?

Part 2—STOP—PRIMARY SURVEY: Are they alive?

Approach and Assess—Are they conscious and can they speak?
Airway—Do they have an open airway?
Breathing—Are they breathing?
Breathing—How well are they breathing?
Circulation—Do they have a pulse?
Circulation—Are they bleeding?
D: Deformity—Are there any obvious deformities?
D: Disability—Is their neck or back at risk of injury?
E: Environment—Can they stay where they are?
E: Everyone Else—Is everyone else high and dry and safe?

Part 3—STOP—SECONDARY SURVEY: How Are They?

- What happened?—the History of Present Illness
- How well are they doing?—Vital Signs
- What are their injuries?—Patient Exam
- What is their past medical history?—AMPLE History
- What is your patient care plan? —SOAPnote

Part 4—STOP—RESCUE SURVEY: Do you need help?

- What is your plan to get help?
- Who is being sent for help? Who is responding? How long will it take for them to arrive?
- What do you need to do to protect the patient while waiting for help to arrive?
- What do you need to do to protect yourselves while waiting for help to arrive?
- Is the scene safe for the group? Is the boat safe?
- Perform on-going assessment; re-SOAP every 15 minutes.

PATIENT ASSESSMENT SYSTEM
in detail

To survey something is to examine it closely and ascertain its condition. In this system of STOP and Survey, the intent is to take the time to STOP and take a deep breath before closely examining and ascertaining the patient's condition. A survey is organized in a logical step-by-step process that allows you to gather the information and respond in an orderly manner.

PART 1: STOP—SCENE SURVEY: Is the Scene Safe?

- Are you OK, and are you going to stay OK?
- Are the others OK, and are they going to stay OK?
- Is the victim of this crisis OK, and are they going to stay OK?
- What happened? What was the mechanism of injury (MOI)?
- How do you safely approach the victim?
- What is your general impression of how serious this is?

To accomplish all this Scene Survey:

Stop. Stand still, take a deep breath, and ask yourself, "Am I OK?" If not, do something about it! Go.

Stop. Tell everyone else to STOP, stand still, take a deep breath and ask themselves, "Am I OK?" If not, do something about it! Don't allow anyone to run off to check the victim or to get help. Go.

Stop. Is the victim OK? First speak or call out to them, even if you cannot see them or get to them. Ask them if they are all right. Hopefully, they will answer; even if they say that they are not all right, at least you know they are alive, have an open airway, are breathing, and have a pulse. Go.

Stop. Ask yourself, "What happened?" "What was the mechanism of injury?" Go.

Stop. Survey the victim's situation. While figuring out how to safely get to them, keep talking to them. Be positive, keep encouraging them, tell them to lie still, that help is on the way. Go.

Stop. As you approach the victim, survey their position. Ask yourself, "Can they stay where they are, or are they in imminent danger and need to be moved?" Go.

Stop. What is your impression of the victim? As you approach the victim (they do not become your patient until you lay your hands on them), develop a general impression of how serious the situation seems to be, based on the position they are lying in, how they look, whether they are conscious, bleeding, etc. Go.

PART 2: STOP—PRIMARY SURVEY:
Are they alive, and are they going to stay alive?

  Approach and Assess—Are they conscious and can they speak?
Airway—Do they have an open airway?

 Breathing—Are they breathing?
Breathing—How well are they breathing?

 Circulation—Do they have a pulse?
Circulation—Are they bleeding?

 Deformity—Are there any obvious deformities?
Disability—Is their neck or back at risk of injury?

Environment—Can they stay where they are?
Everyone Else—How is everyone else in the group doing?

The primary survey is a rapid assessment of all the vital functions necessary to support life: the central nervous system, the respiratory system, and the circulatory system.

- It also takes into consideration how the environment is impacting on the patient.
- If there is a problem, you do not move on to the next step until that problem is solved.
- Each aspect of the primary survey is explored by looking, listening, and feeling.

Look, Listen, & Feel—the keys to the primary survey

Approach and Assess—Are they conscious, and can they speak?

Look—Are they awake; are their eyes open; what position are they lying in?

Listen—Speak to them. Do they speak back?

Feel—What is your general impression of the situation?

- Upon arrival, kneel down next to the patient's head and place a hand on their forehead to hold their head still.
- This not only protects the cervical spine, it also makes physical contact with them, providing "the human touch."
- Continue to speak to them even if they are unconscious.
- The first question you ask is are they conscious or unconscious? If they are conscious, can they speak?
- If they are conscious, ask them to lie still until you have had a chance to check them out.
- Ask the obvious questions: "Are you all right?" "Where does is hurt?" "Do you know what happened?"
- If they are unconscious, you need to make sure that they have an open airway.

Airway—Do they have an open airway?

Look—Is there anything in their airway?

Listen—Can you hear air moving in and out of the airway?

Feel—Can you feel air moving in and out of the airway?

- Lean over your unconscious patient and place your ear in front of their mouth so that you can feel and hear air moving in and out of their airway.
- If they are not breathing, inspect the airway. The most common cause of an obstructed airway is the tongue and position of the head.
- To open the airway, move the head into proper anatomical position. Tilt it slightly back (extension), and gently pull the lower jaw (mandible) forward. This moves the musculature of the tongue forward and opens the airway.
- Again, place you ear over their mouth to make sure that they are breathing.

Breathing—Are they breathing?

Look—Is their chest wall moving as they breathe?

Listen—Can you hear breath sounds?

Feel—Can you feel air moving in and out of their mouth?

- While leaning over, with your ear in front of their mouth, listen to them breathe and make sure air is moving in and out of the airway. Listen to their breath sounds.

- If they are not breathing, give them two full breaths and check to see if they have a pulse. If they have a pulse, continue to give them one full breath every 4–5 seconds until they are breathing on their own.

- If they do not have a pulse, initiate CPR.

Breathing—How well are they breathing?

Look—What is their skin color (are they pale, ashen, blue)?

Listen—Can you hear any adventitious breath sounds such as wheezing, gurgling, or snoring, indicating a partially occluded airway, ?

Feel—Is the chest wall moving appropriately with respirations?

- If they are breathing, listen to see if they are making any adventitious breath sounds such as wheezing, snoring, gurgling, or coughing.

- If any of these sounds are heard, log roll the patient into the recovery position to help clear and maintain an open airway.

- In the recovery position gravity will drain any fluids from the airway and allow the tongue to fall forward opening the airway.

- Never tolerate any adventitious breath sounds as they indicate that the airway is at least partially occluded and the patient is not getting enough oxygen.

- Breathing includes not only whether they are breathing (is air moving in and out of the lungs), but also how well they are breathing.

- Are they breathing often enough and deeply enough to get an adequate supply of oxygen into the lungs and, therefore, into the blood.

- A normal respiratory rate is between 10–30 breaths per minute depending upon age and activity level.

- If they are not taking at least one breath every 6 seconds, 10 breaths per minute, then you need to assist ventilate with at least one full breath every 4–5 seconds.

- If their respiratory rate is greater than 1 breath every 2 seconds or 30 breaths per minute, they are breathing too fast and too shallowly to allow for good air exchange.

- Again assist ventilate them at a rate of one full breath every 4–5 seconds to improve the air exchange in the lungs.

- Now that you know they have an open airway and adequate breathing, check their pulse.

Circulation—Do they have a pulse?

Look—Is their skin pale? Are they cyanotic (bluish)?

Listen—Can you hear a heartbeat?

Feel—Can you feel a carotid pulse?

■ Once you have established that they have an open airway and they are breathing, check a carotid pulse.

■ This is accomplished by placing your 2nd and 3rd fingers over the center of the trachea and drawing your hand towards yourself and into the groove between the trachea and the sternocleidomastoid muscles of the neck. As you gently compress this groove, you will be able to palpate the carotid artery pulse.

■ If they do not have a pulse, initiate CPR. If for some reason you cannot access or feel the carotid pulse, you can place your ear over the left side of the chest to listen for a heartbeat.

Circulation—Are they bleeding?

Look—Is there any active bleeding?

Listen—Can you hear a heartbeat?

Feel—when you cannot see.

■ Along with determining if there is a pulse, you also need to scan the length of their body and look for any signs of obvious bleeding.

■ If there are areas of blood in their clothing or blood pooling on the ground, inspect the area for any source of the bleeding.

■ Slide hands under back, where you cannot see. Pull hands out and look for blood.

■ A minor scrape that is oozing blood can be ignored for now.

■ Your concern is major bleeding from blood that is spurting from the body or rapidly flowing from a wound. This type of bleeding must be controlled.

■ Apply direct pressure to the wound. Remember Body Substance Isolation (BSI) and either put on gloves or create a barrier between you and the body fluid.

Perform a "chunk check" to check for bleeding.

Deformity—Do they have any obvious injuries or deformities?

Look—Do you see any obvious injuries or deformities?

Listen—Where are they complaining of pain?

Feel—Where does it hurt? As you touch them, where can you cause pain?

- This is referred to as a "chunk check."
- Scan the length of the body looking for any obvious deformities like angulated fractures. See if there is anything sticking out of the body that belongs inside or anything sticking into the body that belongs outside.
- Then perform a chunk check by quickly palpating the major parts of the body.
- You want to gently compress the head, the neck, the chest, the abdomen, the pelvis, and the upper legs, feeling for injuries or pain response.
- If you find any injuries, take the time to inspect the area to see if there is something that you need to deal with immediately.

Is their neck or back at risk of injury?

Look—What was the mechanism of injury (MOI)? Can they move their extremities?

Listen—Are they complaining of any neck or back pain?

Feel—Do they have normal sensation in their extremities?

- Upon arrival at the patient's side, you place a hand on the forehead to hold their head still, or you ask someone else to stabilize the cervical spine while you continue the PAS.
- If they are unconscious, or if the mechanism of injury (MOI) indicates possible injury to the spine, continue to immobilize their neck and back.
- Later after completion of the PAS, you will come back and re-examine the spine to see if you can clear it or if you need to continue immobilization of the spine.

Environment—Can they stay where they are?

Look—Where are they lying?

Listen—Are they complaining about being hot, cold, or wet?

Feel—Is their skin warm, dry, cold, or wet?

- Right from the moment you arrive at the patient's side, you have to be asking yourself if they can stay where they are or if they need to be moved.
- Whenever possible, you try to keep them lying still until you can complete the PAS and you have a good idea what the injuries are.
- However, this is not always possible, and you may have to move them without knowing the extent of the injuries.
- If a move is necessary, you have to figure out where they can be safely relocated.
- At a minimum and as soon as possible, get them onto an ensolite pad or other soft, insulating material to protect them from the ground.
- If necessary, surround them with warm insulation or provide shade.
- Eventually they will have to be moved into a shelter to protect them from the weather.

Everyone Else—How is everyone else in the group doing?

Look—How does the rest of the group look?

Listen—Is anyone complaining of being cold, wet, hungry, or thirsty?

Feel—What is the emotional status of the group?

- STOP and consider the whole group.
- How is everyone else doing?
- Is everyone warm and dry and protected from the environment?
- Keep everyone busy.

PART 3: STOP—SECONDARY SURVEY—History of Present Illness, Vital Signs, Patient Exam, AMPLE History, SOAPnote

- What happened?—History of Present Illness
- How well are they?—Vital Signs
- What are their injuries?—Patient Exam
- What is their past medical history?—AMPLE History
- What is our patient care plan?—SOAPnote

Upon completion of the Scene Survey and the Primary Survey, the life-threatening problems have been eliminated or managed. Now you have the luxury of time to move on to the Secondary Survey and answer the question, "How hurt are they?" By taking a set of vital signs, performing a patient exam, and taking an AMPLE history, you will be able to determine the extent and severity of the injuries or illness.

History of Present Illness:

- Onset of injury or illness
- Location of pain or injury
- Quality of pain
- Quantity of pain (0 = no pain; 10 = worst pain ever)

Vital Signs

A person's ability to acquire and utilize oxygen (O_2) is the most important thing. The first responsibility is to make sure the person has an open airway, is breathing, has a pulse, and is not bleeding. Once that is established, you measure and monitor the VITAL SIGNS of the body's major systems in order to determine if a person is getting better, staying the same, or getting worse as a result of injuries, illness, or care provided.

A person can live:

- Weeks without food.
- Days without water.
- Hours in a harsh environment without shelter.
- But only SIX MINUTES without oxygen.

What vital signs tell you:

- How well your patient is doing in response to the injury.
- And how serious the injury is.

What vital signs don't tell you:

- What the specific injury is.

Vital signs set the pace:

- Take a set of vital signs every 5–15 minutes.
- They give you a picture over time of how well your patient is doing.
- They give you confidence that you are doing your job and your patient is doing well.

Vital Signs: By System

Respiratory System (airway and lungs)
The oxygen exchange system: "In with the good air and out with the bad."

- Respiratory Rate: Count the number of breaths per minute—normal: 10-20/minute
- Respiratory Effort: Observe; watch them breathe—normal: no effort
- How hard are they working to breathe?
- Ask them if they feel short of breath, or if they are having a hard time breathing.

Circulatory System (heart, blood vessels, and blood)
Transports the oxygen to every cell in the body: "Do not be still, my beating heart."

- Heart Rate: Find the pulse at the wrist and count it for a minute—normal: 50-100 beats/minute
- Effort: May use a blood pressure (bp) cuff or simply check for pulses—normal: all pulses intact
  - If you get a pulse at the wrist, there is a minimum BP of 90mmHg, enough to perfuse the entire body.
  - If you get a pulse at the femoral artery, there is a minimum BP of 70mmHg, enough to perfuse the vital organs and brain.
  - If you get a pulse at the carotid artery, there is a minimum BP of 60mmHg, enough to perfuse only the brain.

Central Nervous System (brain and spinal cord)
Uses oxygen to survive and thrive and establishes the Level of Consciousness (LOC).

- Monitor LOC with the AVPU scale—normal: awake, alert, oriented x 3

Awake: conscious: how alert are they? —"The lights are on, but is anyone home?"

- Alert and Oriented times one (x1): person—they only know who they are (A&O x 1 = bad).
- Alert and Oriented x 2: place—they know who they are and where they are (A&O x 2 = better).
- Alert and Oriented x 3: time—they know who they are, where they are, the day, week, & year (A&O x 3 = best).

Verbal: unconscious: but do they respond to sound?— "Hello, anyone in there?"

- Speak to them; do they react to hearing their name (attempting to speak, making movement)?
- Do they follow simple commands (blinking, moving a limb)?

Painful: unconscious: but do they respond to pain?—"That's got to hurt."

- Does a knuckle rubbed on their sternum elicit a response (guarding, groaning)?
- Is it an appropriate response to pain?

Unresponsive: unconscious, comatose.

- "No one's home."
- No response to verbal or painful stimuli.

Integumentary System (skin):

The largest organ in the human body, responsible for thermoregulation. If there is limited oxygen, the brain will prioritize and vasoconstrict the peripheral circulation in the skin, shunting the blood away from the skin to vital organs.

Skin color: varies by individual and race.

- Is there perfusion of blood to the skin?
- Check capillary refill.
- Look at the nonpigmented areas of the body: the nail beds, under the eyelids, in the mouth.

Skin temperature and moisture: not too hot, not too cold.

- Touch their skin on the abdomen and in the axilla.
- Are they hot or cold to the touch? Are they dry, wet, or sweaty?

HEALTHY SET OF VITAL SIGNS				
Vital Sign	**Time (0:00)**	**Time (0:15)**	**Time (0:30)**	**Time (0:45)**
RR & Effort	16—no effort	12—no effort	12—no effort	12—no effort
HR & Effort (BP by palp)	80 + radial pulse	72 + radial pulse	60 + radial pulse	60 + radial pulse
LOC	A&O x 3	A&O x 3	A&O x 3	A&O x 3
Skin	warm & moist	warm & moist	warm & moist	warm & moist

VITAL SIGNS IN SHOCK				
Vital Sign	**Time (0:00)**	**Time (0:15)**	**Time (0:30)**	**Time (0:45)**
RR & Effort	16—no effort	12—no effort	20—no effort	30—with effort
HR & Effort (BP by palp)	80 + radial pulse	72 + radial pulse	80 + radial pulse	100 + carotid pulse
LOC	A&O x 3	A&O x 3	A&O x 3 + anxious	A&O x 2 + anxious
Skin	warm & moist	warm & moist	pale & cool	pale, cool, & clammy

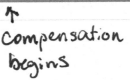

↑ compensation begins

Patient Exam—The principles of a thorough search for trouble

- Hands-on, head-to-toe exam that locates the injuries.
- Done in much the same way as a good massage.
- One person does the entire exam.
- Start at the head; then do: neck—chest—abdomen—legs—arms—back.
- Talk with the patient; explain what you are doing.
- If they complain of pain, ask where it hurts.
- Avoid unnecessary movement.
- History of Present Illness—get a thorough history of what happened.

Principles of the Patient Exam—you are trying to discover all possible injuries by:

INSPECTION: Look for bleeding & wounds, impaled objects, deformities.

CIRCULATION: Check all four extremities for pulses.

C

COMPARISON: Check symmetry of body parts.

SENSATION: Check all four extremities for sensation.

S

PALPATION: Is there tenderness in muscles, bones, or joints?

MOTION: Check all four extremities for the ability to move.

M

HEAD: Inspect scalp, face, eyes, nose, mouth, ears.

NECK: Palpate cervical spine, inspect trachea.

CHEST: Palpate clavicles, shoulder, and compress the rib cage.

ABDOMEN: Compress the abdomen in the center.

PELVIS: Compress the pelvis front to back and laterally.

LEGS: Palpate the muscles and ask patient to flex the joints.

ARMS: Palpate the muscles and ask patient to flex their joints.

BACK: Palpate the length of the back.

AMPLE History

Everyone has a past medical history that others may not be aware of. This medical history can be very important and can be a factor in providing proper medical care. Use the simple mnemonic of AMPLE to remind yourself of the appropriate questions to ask your patients about their medical history.

Allergies
- To medications, foods, insects, etc.
- What happens and how is it treated?

Medications
- What medications are they taking (both prescription and over-the-counter)?
- Have they taken their meds today? How often and how much?

Previous Injury or Illness
- Any recent or past injury or illness that could contribute to the current problem?

Last Input and Output
- When was the last time they ate or drank?
- What did they eat and drink?
- When was the last time they voided or had a bowel movement?

Events leading up to the crisis
- What led up to or occurred just prior to the critical event?

Allergies?

Medications?

History?

Last in, last out

What happened??

SOAPnote

SOAPNOTE

Subjective: age, sex, mechanism of injury (MOI), chief complaint(C/C): 22 year old male. Slipped and fell on wet deck - slid across deck into closed hatch and is now complaining of pain in right ankle and right knee.

Objective: vital signs, patient exam, AMPLE history:

Vital Signs							
TIME	13:30	13:45	14:00	14:45			
LOC oriented x ?	A+O×2	A+O×2	A+O×2				
RR & effort	20	16	12				
HR & effort	88	72	60				
Skin C, T, M	P/c/c	P/c/c	P/c/c				

Patient Exam: Describe locations of pain, tenderness & injuries: 22 year old male who appears cold. Skin is pale, cool, and clammy to the touch. He answers questions accurately but slowly - very apathetic - shivering slightly. Positive for pain on palpation of R. Hand, R. Knee, R. ankle. Abrasion on palm R hand. Full ROM & CSM q R hand and wrist r. Right knee is stable in all planes - no swelling, but tenderness. R. Ankle is swollen and tender. There is crepitation w/ ankle motion. Neurologically intact. Spine is cleared.

Allergies: Penicillin, Sulfa, Codeine.

Medications: Sudafed, Albuterol Inhaler

Past pertinent medical history: Seasonal allergies, exercise induced asthma.

Last in and out: had lunch at 12:30. Cheese, bread, brownie, water.

Events leading up to accident:
Was on foredeck overhauling jib sheets.

Assessment: problem list:
1. Possible fractured right ankle
2. Pain in R. Knee
3. Abrasion R. Hand -
4. Hypothermia

Plan: plan for each problem on the problem list: Splinted R. Knee - position q comfort w/ blanket.
1. R. Ankle splinted w/ PFD and duct tape.
2. Abrasion cleaned and bandaged
3. Wet clothing removed and hypothermia wrapped, oral sweet fluids.
4. MONITOR - How often do you plan to monitor the patient? Every 15 min for improvement of Hypothermia. Will continue - sweet - warm fluids.

©2007 SOLO

27

PATIENT ASSESSMENT CHECK LIST

SCENE SIZE-UP:

- ☐ Is the SCENE SAFE?
- ☐ Is the PATIENT SAFE?
- ☐ BSI? *Body Substance Isolation (put on gloves, mask)*

- ☐ MOI – Mechanism of Injury
- ☐ GI – General Impression
- ☐ Self – take care of yourself

PRIMARY SURVEY:

- ☐ Is the patient CONSCIOUS?
- ☐ Do they have an OPEN AIRWAY?
- ☐ Are they BREATHING?
- ☐ Are they BLEEDING? / CIRCULAT
- ☐ Do they have a PULSE?
- ☐ Are there any serious injuries on the CHUNK CHECK?
- ☐ Do they need to be MOVED?
- ☐ Do they need to be DE-CRUMPLED?
- ☐ Do you need to protect them from the ENVIRONMENT?

Aairway Breathing Circulation Deformity Environ / everyone else

SECONDARY SURVEY—VITAL SIGNS:

- ☐ What is their RESPIRATORY RATE & EFFORT?
- ☐ What is their HEART RATE & EFFORT?
- ☐ What is their LEVEL OF CONSCIOUSNESS?
- ☐ What is their SKIN COLOR, TEMPERATURE, & MOISTURE?

SECONDARY SURVEY—PATIENT EXAM:

- [ ] HEAD—scalp, face, eyes, nose, mouth

- [ ] NECK—spine, trachea

- [ ] CHEST—clavicles, shoulders, ribs

- [ ] ABDOMEN—compress the abdomen

- [ ] PELVIS—compress the pelvis, anterior/posterior and lateral

- [ ] LEGS—circulation, sensation, and motion

- [ ] ARMS—circulation, sensation, and motion

- [ ] BACK—log roll and palpate the length of the spine

SECONDARY SURVEY—AMPLE HISTORY:

- [ ] ALLERGY—allergy to drugs, foods, insects, etc.

- [ ] MEDS—prescription and non-prescription drugs

- [ ] PREVIOUS—significant past medical history, surgeries, etc.

- [ ] LAST—last intake & last output

- [ ] EVENT—events leading up to this crisis

SOAPNOTE—RECORD VITAL INFORMATION:
ON-GOING ASSESSMENT

- [ ] Record patient data.

- [ ] Re-SOAP every 15 minutes.

MAKE A RESCUE PLAN

Part 4: STOP—Rescue Survey—how to get help

The Patient Assessment System has been completed. You now combine the patient's condition with the group's condition and determine if you need help from rescuers.

Patient's condition:
- [ ] Continuously monitor the patient's condition.
- [ ] Re-**SOAP** every 15 minutes.

    S: are they hungry, thirsty, in pain, need to go to the bathroom?

    O: take and record a complete set of vital signs, check all splints and bandages for circulation.

    A: is assessment the same?

    P: is the plan the same?

Group's condition:
- [ ] How well is each individual in the group doing: hungry, thirsty, anxious?
- [ ] How well-prepared is the group to stay aboard? Or on a river trip, to bivouac on shore.

Decisions:
- [ ] Do you need to evacuate the patient or can you all go on?
- [ ] If evacuation is needed, get help.
- [ ] While waiting for rescue—Is the boat secure; what is the condition of the rest of the crew? Is the situation stable?

Sending for help:
- [ ] Can you radio for help? Do you have cell reception?
- [ ] Who do you call? Do you have other ways to signal for help?
- [ ] Prepare a SOAP note to radio out, or to go with the patient.
- [ ] Prepare a list of the remaining group and how well-prepared they are to stay with the boat, or on the trip.
- [ ] Prepare to give your exact position, in latitude and logitude, as well as using local landmarks.

While waiting for help to arrive:
- [ ] Keep spirits up, be positive, reassure, make sure everyone has something to do.
- [ ] Create light and warmth; keep everyone warm and dry.
- [ ] Make yourselves big, easy to find. Use signal flags and flares.
- [ ] Continuously monitor your patient and the other members of your group.

International signal flag W for Whiskey
"Require Medical Assistance"

PATIENT LIFTING & MOVING TECHNIQUES

When an injury occurs, it is important to keep the wounded person lying still, as they may not know how seriously they are hurt. This can be made more difficult on a heaving deck or on a moving boat in a large sea, or in small boats in white-water.

The very first component of patient care you will need to provide is to safely lift or move the patient to another location. This is to protect them from further harm or protect them from the environment. This may occur anytime during the Initial Assessment, Primary Survey, or Secondary Survey.

 Are they in immediate danger from falling overboard, or from thrashing gear?

 Are they lying in water?

 Are they lying on a cold or slippery surface?

 Are they lying on sharp debris, or in danger from unsecured objects that could fall on them?

 Are they generally in harm's way?

If your patient is in harm's way, you are also in harm's way. One victim is enough.

When possible, try to perform a patient exam or chunk check before moving your patient so you have an idea of what the injuries are.

Personal Safety Precautions:

 Know your own strength and physical limitations.

 Work together—get as many hands on the patient as possible; many hands make light work.

The cardinal rule of moving hurt people...

It is always safe to move someone from the position of injury to the position of function.

...but

Avoid flexion of the head and neck.

    ■ May move the head & neck into neutral position, but do not flex forward.

Avoid rotation of the pelvis out of alignment with the shoulders.

    ■ May line up the shoulders and the pelvis, but do not rotate out of alignment.

POSITIONS:

SUPINE: Lying flat on your back.

PRONE: Lying flat on your chest & stomach.

RECOVERY POSITION: 3/4 prone position used to maintain the airway.

The recovery position.

When lifting, use proper body mechanics:

    ■ Lift with your legs.

    ■ Keep your back straight and your butt down.

    ■ Try not to overreach or twist.

    ■ Keep the weight as close to your body as possible.

    ■ Use assists such as blankets, rain flies, or ensolite pads.

Always lift properly.

LIFTING AND MOVING:

LOG ROLL: Keeping the head, shoulders, and pelvis in line, roll the patient onto their side.

MOVE AS A UNIT: With many hands on, move the person as if they were frozen stiff.

DRAGS: Drag them by their clothing or on a pad.

TRANSFERS & CARRIES: With many hands, pick them up and walk:

ONE-PERSON: Roll onto a pad to drag.

TWO-PERSON: May be able to carry or drag.

MANY PERSONS: Much easier, many hands on.

SHOCK

A condition in which the cardiovascular system fails to provide sufficient circulation to every part of the body causing tissues to eventually suffer from a lack of oxygen.

The CARDIOVASCULAR SYSTEM consists of:

- Heart—pumps the blood.
- Blood vessels—carry and distribute the blood.
- Blood—carries the oxygen.

Shock is a compensatory mechanism designed to keep the brain well-oxygenated during times of cardiovascular insufficiency by:

- Vasoconstricting the peripheral circulation, thus pooling blood into the body core,
- Increasing the heart rate, which sends more blood to the brain, and
- Increasing respiratory rate to maximize the amount of oxygen in the blood.

- These COMPENSATORY MECHANISMS occur whenever the BRAIN perceives a threat or crisis, real or not, and puts the cardiovascular system on ALERT STATUS.
  The ALERT STATUS is transient and self-correcting. SHOCK is the compensatory mechanism caused by failure of the cardiovascular system in its effort to maintain circulation and thus oxygen to the brain.
- In SHOCK the compensatory mechanism prioritizes the blood flow from the heart to the lungs to the brain. The only other organs involved are the liver and kidneys.
- Once injuries are properly treated, the shock condition or Alert Status should cease and the vital signs return to normal. If not, the person is in life-threatening shock.
- Initially shock status is a life-saving condition that preserves blood flow to the brain, but SHOCK KILLS if it continues for too long. You have to find the underlying cause.

Causes of shock:

- HYPOVOLEMIC: **LOW VOLUME** caused by decreased blood volume due to blood loss or dehydration from sweating, diarrhea, vomiting, or a burn.
- CARDIOGENIC: **LOW FLOW** caused by pump failure, i.e. a heart attack.
- NEUROGENIC: **LOW PRESSURE** caused by vasodilation, a loss of vascular tone, that results in increased vascular space, from spinal cord injury and acute allergic reaction to life-threatening infection, "blood poisoning," or septic shock.

SIGNS & SYMPTOMS

Individuals in shock are not quite "there."

- They are distant.
- They stare off into space or may be unconscious.
- They may not know you are there.
- They may not feel pain or respond to pain.
- They may have an obvious wound or injury that they ignore.
- They may try to walk on a broken leg or use a broken arm.
- They do not know how seriously they are injured.
- They may have a sense of impending doom.

- LOC: restless, anxious, may be disoriented,
- RR: rapid & shallow (increased respiratory rate, more oxygen),
- HR: rapid & weak & thready (increased heart rate, to deliver more blood to the brain),
- SKIN: pale, cool, clammy (due to the vasoconstriction of the capillaries in the skin),
- May collapse; typically nauseous and may vomit.

CARE & TREATMENT:

- ✔ **AIRWAY, AIRWAY, AIRWAY.**
- ✔ Control **BLEEDING** to minimize blood loss.
- ✔ **FIND AND TREAT THE UNDERLYING CAUSE.**
- ✔ Treat all injuries to minimize pain.
- ✔ Keep them lying flat in a position of comfort; may elevate the legs.
- ✔ Protect from the environment; maintain body temperature. — *keep 'em warm & dry*
- ✔ Monitor vital signs, reassure, & get help.

— *NOTES*—

CHAPTER TWO

TRAUMA: MUSCULOSKELETAL INJURIES
Strains, Sprains, and Broken Bones

TRAUMA: MUSCULOSKELETAL INJURIES

MUSCULOSKELETAL SYSTEM (BONES, MUSCLES, TENDONS, LIGAMENTS)

When your musculoskeletal system is working properly, this framework of bones, muscles, tendons, ligaments, and cartilage is what holds you up and allows you to move and function.

WHAT THEY DO:

■ **BONES** provide the structure to which everything attaches. Bones also store calcium and produce blood cells in the bone marrow.

■ **CARTILAGE** acts as a lubricated pad between bones so that your joints can flex or rotate smoothly. Cartilage also provides support for muscle in areas where more flexibility than bone is needed (like your ears).

■ **SYNOVIAL FLUID** is the lubricant in the joint space and is produced by the synovial lining of the joint capsule.

■ **MUSCLES** are like bundles of bungee cords. They contract or relax in response to signals sent from your brain through your central nervous system, which flexes your joints and allows you to move. Muscles also provide some padding and protection for nerve-bundles, arteries, and veins.

■ **LIGAMENTS** are like nylon cords and attach bones to other bones. They maintain proper range of motion.

■ **TENDONS** are ties connecting muscle to bone. They span joints and allow for movement.

MUSCULOSKELETAL SYSTEM FUNCTIONS:

- Movement.
- Protection of underlying structures.
- Calcium storage.
- Blood cell production (Hematopoiesis).
- Heat production.
- Cosmesis (your muscles and bones determine how you look).

ANATOMICAL POSITION

When describing the position of parts of the body in relationship to each other, parts that are farther away from the core of the body are described as "DISTAL" and parts that are closer to the core of the body are "PROXIMAL."

TYPES OF MUSCULOSKELETAL INJURIES:

- Sprains and Strains—twisting and pulling damage to the supporting structure of joints (ligaments, muscles, and tendons) are by far the most common backcountry injuries.
- Fractures—breaks of the hard outer layer of bone can be particularly dangerous because the sharp ends of the bones can cause damage to the surrounding muscle, nerves, and blood vessels.

SPRAINS & STRAINS:

Signs and Symptoms:

✓ Generalized pain around a joint, no point tenderness.

✓ Pain with movement of the joint.

✓ Minimal pain with weight-bearing.

✓ Swelling can be dramatic.

✓ May become discolored over time, "black and blue" (ecchymosis).

Treatment: the primary goal is to minimize swelling by using RICE:

✓ Rest: stop and sit down; this slows circulation.

✓ Ice: causes vasoconstriction, decreasing circulation—ice, snow, or wet.

✓ Compression: decreases circulation and room for swelling; the less it swells the faster it will heal.

✓ Elevation: decreases circulation.

✓ Immobilize & support the affected joint.

FRACTURES:

◼ Bones are made up of a hard outer layer of compact bone and an inner soft area of bone marrow.

◼ A fracture occurs when enough force is exerted against a bone to break the outer compact bone.

EVALUATING A MUSCULOSKELETAL INJURY:

SPRAIN (+/oR) FRACTURE

	SPRAIN	FRACTURE
Look—What do you see when you examine the injury?		
◼ Do they have normal movement and function?	Usually	No
◼ Are they guarding the injury?	Slightly	Yes
◼ Do you see any deformity or angulations?	No	Yes
◼ Do you see any discoloration or swelling?	Maybe	Yes
Listen—Talk to the patient; what do they say?		
◼ What happened?		
◼ What was the Mechanism Of Injury (MOI)?		
◼ Where does it hurt?		
◼ Did they feel anything snap, crack, or pop?	Maybe	Usually
Feel—What do you feel when you examine the injury?		
◼ Is there good Circulation, Sensation, and Motion (CSM)?	Usually	Maybe
◼ Is there point tenderness?	No	Yes
◼ Is there crepitation (the sound of broken bones grinding)?	No	Yes

Muscle under normal tension

Fracture

If the Mechanism of Injury indicates a possible fracture, treat as such.

WHEN IN DOUBT, SPLINT!

THE PRINCIPLES OF SPLINTING:

 Can the injury be immobilized in the position found? **Check circulation.**

⌐ IF NO PULSE IN extremity

 If not, pull <u>traction-in-line</u> to slowly and gently move the extremity into proper anatomical *) 10-15 min.* alignment. This establishes and maintains circulation distal to the site of the injury.

 Create a rigid but **well-padded** splint (well-insulated in winter); fill all voids.

 Immobilize the **entire extremity**, including the joint above and below the site of the injury.

 Monitor all splints; check C/S/M distal to the site of the injury every fifteen minutes.

SPLINTING PROCEDURES:

Improvise cervical collar:
- Used to protect neck.
- Soft, conforms to neck.
- Warm.
- Comfortable.

Arm sling & swathe—uses:
- Dislocated shoulder.
- Fractured clavicle.
- Fractured humerus.
- Fractured forearm, wrist, hand.
- Elbow injury.
- Fractured ribs. *~ arm acts as the splint*

Forearm splint:

- Rigid splint with sticks, pack stays, etc. used with arm sling and swathe.
- Sam Splint used with arm sling and swathe.

— don't wrap

Improvised lower leg & ankle splint:

- Rigid splint with sticks, poles, skis, etc.
- Ensolite pad splint.

Improvised knee splint:

- Splint knee in position of comfort (30^0 +/-).
- Place padding in the hollow behind the knee.

Sprained ankle bandage:

- To splint a fractured ankle or support a sprained ankle.

43

SPINAL CORD INJURY MANAGEMENT:

■ Pre-hospital personnel are trained to treat all possible spinal cord injuries based on the Mechanism Of Injury (MOI) as well as symptoms and complaints.

■ It is important in the marine/wilderness environment for rescuers to recognize a possible back injury based on MOI, but it is equally important that they be able to rule it out or "clear the spine" by a proper history and physical exam in order to avoid an unnecessary litter evacuation.

■ Spinal assessment—to clear the spine—is not performed until after the patient assessment system has been completed and it is appropriate to evaluate and potentially clear the spine of any possible injury.

Method of clearing the spine: Patient must meet all of these criteria to clear the spine.

12 hrs.

■ Patient must be sober, conscious, coherent, and oriented x 3, in person, place, & time.

■ Patient has no painful distracting injuries (e.g. fractured femur, compound fracture, burn).

■ Patient does not complain of any pain the entire length of the back.

■ Patient does not have radiating pain, paresthesias (tingling), paralysis, or numbness in any of their extremities.

■ Patient has intact sensation and motion in all four extremities unless local injury.

■ Patient has no tenderness on physical exam along the entire length of the back.

■ Without assistance, the patient is able to flex, extend, and rotate neck, upper, and lower back without pain or discomfort, and this movement is symmetrical without locking sensation or limited range of motion.

■ You can always move the patient into proper anatomical position.

C7

T12

L5

sacrum & coccyx

SPINAL CORD INJURY MANAGEMENT:

- It is more important to know how to move an injured person, to protect them from further injury than it is to know how to backboard them.
- Cervical spine is at risk with flexion; do not lift head.
- Lumbar spine is at risk with rotation; keep shoulders, and hips aligned.
- Lifting and moving techniques were discussed with Patient Assessment.

Cervical Collars:

- You can improvise very comfortable and immobilizing soft blanket and horseshoe collars out of materials such as a pile jacket, blanket, or ensolite pad. They provide support, comfort, and warmth.

Backboards:

- Backboards or litters are only used by rescue teams for transport.
- While waiting for help to arrive, simply keep the patient still, comfortable, and warm.
- Protect them from the cold or hot surface.
- Remember not to flex the neck! Keep the spine straight by log rolling the patient.

Head Injuries

The potential for head injuries on a boat are greater than in many other outdoor activities.

What to consider in the event of a head injury:

- Did the patient lose consciousness—even momentarily?
- Is there bleeding or fluid coming from the patient's ears?
- Is the patient at all disoriented?
- Do they have a lot of head pain as a result of the injury?
- Is there injury or danger to eyes, mouth or teeth?

If the answer to any of these questions is "yes," then you need to evacuate the patient immediately.

Remember:

- In the event of a head injury, evacuation IS the treatment.

- In the case of a head injury, the clock is running. The best treatment involves getting the patent to definitive care with as little delay as possible.

Broken Or Dislocated Digits:

Between the number of obstacles on a boat deck like ring-bolts, stanchions, standing rigging, and blocks, and the lines that run through those blocks, there are multiple opportunities for broken or dislocated fingers or toes.

HOW TO REDUCE A DISLOCATED DIGIT:

Make sure that your hands and theirs are dry, as you are going to need a good grip.
Apply traction-in-line (TIL) and slowly increase the effort of traction.

As you are applying TIL, push down on the elevated side and up on the depressed side. With this technique, the joint will snap back into place.
Check circulation, sensation, and motion (CSM) before splinting the finger in position of comfort.
Position of comfort for the fingers is in a partially flexed position, as if the hand was gripping a glass of water or soda can.

SPLINTING A FRACTURED FINGER:

Fractures of the digits can be obvious with deformity at the site of the fracture, or they can be subtle with little more than swelling and discoloration, ecchymosis, at the fracture site.

If there is a fracture, the patient will find it painful to try to flex or extend the digit, and there will be pain with gentle in-line traction or compression when examining the digit.

HOW TO SPLINT A FRACTURED FINGER OR TOE:

If the fracture is angulated, apply gentle TIL and slowly move the digit into proper anatomical position.

Splint the finger in position of comfort.
Always try to splint the fingers in a partially flexed position as if the fingers were wrapped around a can of soda.

HOW TO BUDDY TAPE TOES:

Buddy taping works very well for toes and can be used for support until the injury has healed.
This is accomplished by placing some soft padding between the two toes and taping them together so that the good digit can support the injured one.
The patient needs to wear stiff soled shoes to support the fracture site until healed.

— NOTES—

CHAPTER THREE

ENVIRONMENTAL EMERGENCIES & SURVIVAL SKILLS

How To Survive and Thrive in the World

ENVIRONMENTAL EMERGENCIES AND SURVIVAL SKILLS:

Before you examine environmental threats, it is critical that you understand how your body reacts to changes in your environment. You have characteristics that make you both wonderfully suited to your environment and yet terribly susceptible to its fluctuations.

THE HUMAN ANIMAL

- Humans are a true tropical animal—an essentially hairless being with sweat glands.
- You are warm-blooded and, through metabolism, are constantly generating heat.
- Your skin is your largest organ, accounting for about 10% of your body's weight; it is the primary organ of thermoregulation.
- You have one of the most sensitive and efficient regulatory mechanisms on the planet for surviving and thriving in the heat; it is designed to keep your brain at a relatively constant temperature.
- You sweat, and the evaporation of water from your skin cools the blood in the skin and, thus, the systemic circulation. Fur-covered mammals and birds pant, which evaporates water out of the airways, thus cooling their blood in the pulmonary circulation.
- You do not survive because of physical prowess but by your mental prowess.
- You have only rudimentary defensive mechanisms to protect you in the cold (e.g. frostbite only numbs us; it does not produce a painful warning).

Because of these characteristics, humans are perfectly suited to life in the tropics where the ability to shed heat is more important than the ability to retain it. However, as populations grew and moved north or south of the tropics, this ability became a hinderance because they often found themselves cooling off faster than they could generate or maintain heat, resulting in hypothermia, risk of frostbite, and impaired mental function. "A cold brain is a dumb brain."

THE HUMAN BRAIN

- In order for your brain to function normally, it needs a constant supply of oxygen and glucose, and a consistent temperature between 97^0 and 104^0F.

- Anatomy and Function: You can think of the brain like an onion with each layer that is added on being a layer of increased function or intelligence.

- The **Brainstem** is at the top of the spinal cord in the center of the brain. It controls the functions that maintain life from second-to-second ("reptilian brain"). Found in this structure are:
    - The respiratory center that controls breathing.
    - The cardiovascular center that controls heart rate and blood pressure.
    - The thermoregulatory center that maintains core temperature.
    - The reticuloactivating center that maintains level of consciousness.

- The **Primitive Brain** or **limbic brain** surrounds the brainstem. It controls the functions that allow you to survive day-to-day and as a species ("primitive brain"):
    - The need to procreate (sex drive).
    - Defensive posturing, primitive aggressive reflexes.

- The **Higher Brain** or **cerebral cortex** is what makes you human. It controls the functions that allow you to survive, strive, and thrive:
    - Gross motor coordination.
    - Fine motor coordination.
    - Reasoning, problem-solving, and judgment.

- When you impair the brain, it loses functions from the most advanced layer, the outermost layer, in. So you lose judgment and problem-solving first and the ability to breathe last.

cerebral cortex

limbic brain

cerebellum

brainstem

THERMOREGULATION: BALANCING THE TEMPERATURE

HEAT PRODUCTION:

- Basal metabolism is the constant biochemistry that produces heat.
- You burn glucose to produce the heat to drive other chemical reactions.
- Exercise, muscle activity, produces heat.
- Voluntary or involuntary shivering can increase heat production 5x's.

HEAT CONSERVATION:

- Vasoconstriction of the blood vessels in the skin.
- Piloerection—hair standing on end.
- Cessation of sweating.
- Posturing—assuming positions to conserve body heat.

PHYSICS OF HEAT LOSS: (LAWS OF THERMODYNAMICS):

- Conduction   0%–40% depending upon the type of solid material.
- Convection   0%–40% depending upon air penetration.
- Radiation   5%–80% depending upon surrounding temperature.
- Evaporation   0%–90% depending upon vapor pressure & moisture .

conduction

convection

radiation

According to the NASBLA*, "A person immersed in cold water will lose body heat 25 times faster than someone not immersed in water". (This assumes water and air temperatures are the same.)

evaporation

*NASBLA is the National Association of State Boating Law Administrators.

NUTRITION:

Nutritional Requirements: the average person needs about 2500 calories/day.

- Carbohydrate: 4cal/gram 60% (200–400 grams/day = 1200–1600 cal/day).
- Protein: 4cal/gram 30% (30–55 grams/day = 120–220 cal/day).
- Fat: 9cal/gram 10% (20–60 grams/day = 180–540 cal/day).

Number of calories required varies with activity:

- Normal daily activity: 2000–2500 calories/day.
- Winter outdoor sports: 3000–4000 calories/day.
- High altitude activities: 4000–6000 calories/day.

HYDRATION:

Hydration Requirements: the average person needs about two liters of fluid per day.

Normal water losses per day:	Normal Temp	Hot Temp	Heavy Exercise
Skin (moisture loss)	350ml	350ml	350ml
Respiration (breathing)	250ml	350ml	650ml
Sweating	100ml	1400ml	**5000ml**
Urination	1400ml	1200ml	500ml
Defecation	100ml	100ml	100ml
TOTALS	**2200ml**	**3400ml**	**6600ml**

Water requirements will vary with activity, sweat output, and altitude.

- Exertional sweat loss is 1–3 liters/hour for up to 4 hours without replacement.
- Altitude has a very low vapor pressure; you will lose about 1cup/hour via respirations. (24 cups/24 hrs., 6 quarts or liters/24 hrs., 1½ gallons every 24 hrs.)

You have to be able to make pure potable (drinkable) water.

- In a salt-water environment, how big is your fresh water tank? Do you have a reverse osmosis watermaker?
- If you have access to fresh, water do you have a method to treat it? Potable water—chemicals, filtering, boiling.

HYPOTHERMIA:

Hypothermia: Is a lowering of the body's core temperature to a level where normal brain & muscle function are impaired. Remember the onion analogy. As the body cools, function is lost from the most advanced layer down.

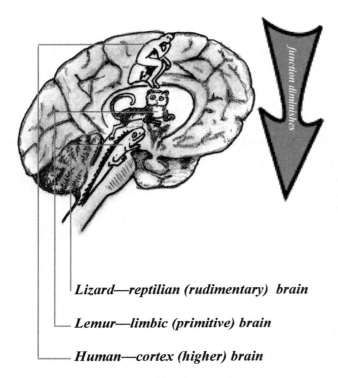

Lizard—reptilian (rudimentary) brain

Lemur—limbic (primitive) brain

Human—cortex (higher) brain

function diminishes

- People suffering from hypothermia do "mindless" things like leaving food, water, and shelter behind.
- Hypothermia is insidious in that you cannot detect the danger signs in yourself.
- Even though the signs and symptoms of hypothermia may be very obvious when exhibited in others, when you become hypothermic, you think everything is fine.

The body's defensive reaction to cooling off: Losing more heat than it produces.

- Skin: peripheral vasoconstriction to decrease blood flow to the skin and thus decrease heat loss.
- Involuntary shivering: uncoordinated muscle activity to produce heat.
- Increased basal metabolism: burn glucose to produce heat—rate may increase 5 fold.
- Behavioral: put on warm clothes, seek out shelter, warmth, protection.

There is no warning of impending doom:

- You do not have a cold center in your brain that warns you that you are becoming hypothermic.
- You get cold, you get dumb, you get lost, you get hurt, you cause problems.

Stages of Hypothermia:

98.6F	Normal
97F	The brain falters, judgment fails, protective & survival instincts decrease. At this point you are in trouble, as you do not take measures to protect yourself. As temperature decreases, mental abilities decrease.
96F	Shivering begins, a constant fine motor tremor. You cannot stop it. It interferes with coordinated muscle activity.
94F	You shiver harder; coordination is failing; you begin tripping and falling.
92F	Shivering is intense; you are unable to walk.
90F	Shivering is convulsive; you assume the fetal position; you are unable to talk.
86F	and below: The "Metabolic Icebox;" you are unconscious, ashen gray; you may appear pulseless and breathless.

According to the NASBLA, if water temperature and air temperature are the same; a person immersed in cold water will lose body heat 25 times faster than someone not immersed in water.

Prevention: **Know your enemy and be prepared for wet, wind, & cold.**

☑ Carry and use rain gear: pants and jacket.

☑ Wear fabrics that stay warm when wet.

☑ Snack often on foods high in quick-burning carbohydrates/glucose.

☑ Stay WELL-HYDRATED.

☑ On a river or inshore, carry bivouac gear and know how to use it.

☑ Be attentive to yourself, companions and the environment.

Treatment: **Remove the patient from immediate danger & further exposure.**

☑ Create or seek out shelter.

☑ Get DRY & keep DRY.

☑ Give lots of warm, sweet liquids (JELL-O with <u>sugar</u>) if conscious.

☑ Insulate with hypothermia wrap.

The preferred method for field rewarming of a hypothermic patient involves two principles: Helping the patient to continue to generate body heat and preventing the patient from losing that heat to the environment.

One of the best ways to generate body heat is to feed fuel to the furnace. Foods like powdered JELL-O dissolved in warm water are easy for most patients to take and can provide the needed caloric energy for the patient to start generating more heat.

HYPOTHERMIA: THE HYPOWRAP— BUILDING THE HUMAN BURRITO

Once refueling has started, the next step is to stop the patient from losing body heat and create an environment that allows them to store the heat they are producing. The Hypowrap provides an excellent environment for rewarming and protects the patient from the weather.

- Get the patient dry and keep them dry.
- Remove any wet clothing from the patient.
- Reinsulate them with **DRY MATERIAL**—clothing, sleeping bags.
- Place them on an insulating layer such as a dry foam pad.
- Surround the patient with a windproof, waterproof layer—plastic sheeting, tarp.
- Monitor their condition and take appropriate actions as conditions change.

PRINCIPLES OF TREATING HYPOTHERMIA

- Protect from the environment.
- Stop the heat loss.
- Stoke the fire—feed and hydrate.
- Insulate to minimize heat loss.
- If unconscious, do not attempt to feed.
- Make sure everyone in the group is warm and dry.

Prepare a base of protective and insulating material. Windproof and waterproof outer layer with insulating layer (ensolite).

Add lots of dry insulation.

Place patient inside. Double-protect feet and head.

Wrap securely and monitor condition.

FROSTBITE:

Frostbite: **Is a localized cooling and/or freezing of tissue caused by the shunting of blood away from cold areas of the body.**

Superficial: description **and treatment:**

- 1st degree: "frostnip"—numb, soft, cold, pallor.
- 2nd degree: numb, soft, cold, pallor, pain on thawing, and formation of clear fluid-filled or blood-filled bleb.
- Field rewarm using skin-to-skin contact.
- Never massage, rub with snow, or use an external heat source.
- If a bleb forms, protect the area and evacuate the patient.
- Beware of refreezing which can happen quickly and will cause much greater tissue damage.

Deep: description **and treatment:**

- 3rd degree: numb, cold, white, and rock hard; massive blebs form when thawed; extreme pain during thawing.
- Protect the area and evacuate the patient.
- DO NOT field rewarm (once thawed the area is useless and excruciatingly painful).

2nd degree with blebs

1st degree

3rd degree

Prevention: Keep the whole body warm.

✔ If your feet are cold, put on a hat.

✔ Eat & drink to maintain a constant energy/heat production—maintain blood sugar.

✔ STAY DRY! CARRY AND USE RAIN GEAR—TOPS & BOTTOMS.

✔ Pack extra socks, hats, mittens, or any clothing that is likely to get wet.

✔ Wear wool or pile. (Cotton is warm only as long as it is dry.)

✔ Do not drink alcohol or use tobacco.

✔ Avoid tight clothing and clothing that will hold water against the skin for extended periods of time, such as neoprene gloves and neoprene booties.

✔ Keep an eye on each other.

HEAT INJURIES:

Heat Exhaustion:

- Not a life-threatening emergency. Heat-exhausted patients often recover without care.
- Usually occurs in people who are not acclimatized to heat.
- Cause: A combination of salt and water loss secondary to sweating = dehydration.
- May be associated with heat cramps.
- Heat exhaustion can progress to heat stroke.

Signs & Symptoms: Typically complain of mild headache, dizziness, and nausea.

- Skin: pale, cool, clammy.
- LOC: may be normal or slightly anxious.
- Pulse: slightly increased, but BP is normal.
- Resp.: may be normal or slightly increased with normal effort.

Treatment:

- Rest in a cool place in the shade.
- Replace lost fluid & salt—1 teaspoon salt + 2 tablespoons (8 teaspoons) of sugar in 1 liter/quart of water. This is an oral rehydration solution (ORS). ORS can also be used to replace fluids lost from diarrhea, vomiting, fever (sweating), or burns. Other ORS are:
    - Commercial: Gatorade
    - Fruits: oranges, melons, lemons, and limes, either eaten or juiced

one teaspoon salt

plus two
tablespoons sugar

plus one
liter water

EQUALS
TREATMENT

Heat Stroke:

A true LIFE-THREATENING EMERGENCY! The patient will die without immediate care!

Two Causes:

- One: The person has become dehydrated by sweating out fluid faster than they replace it. As their sweating mechanism fails, their body temperature goes up rapidly.

- Two: With a hot day and high humidity, the sweat cannot evaporate off their skin fast enough to cool them. (Exertional heatstroke).

Signs & Symptoms:

- Skin: RED, HOT, DRY (50%); OTHER 50% ARE WET.
- Temp.: $105°F +$, maximum survivable core temperature is $107°F$.
- LOC: Disoriented, confused, combative, hallucinating, eventually coma & death.
- Pulse: Rapid and full; BP may be elevated.
- Resp.: Full and deep.

Treatment: This is one of the few conditions where immediate treatment is essential.

- REMOVE FROM HEAT & SUN.
- COOL IMMEDIATELY by soaking with water & fanning to accelerate evaporation.
- Hydrate if possible.
- Vigorously massage limbs.
- Beware of shivering—shivering produces heat.
- Transport immediately to the hospital.

Prevention: Stay out of the hot noonday sun.

- Hydrate or die.
- Stay hydrated & eat salty foods.
- Keep your head covered; wear cotton that will hold moisture which cools the skin.
- Beware of warning signs: feel hot, feel dry, can't pee.

buzzard

agua

hombre

saguaro cactus

MARINE BITES AND STINGS

Three Primary Concerns:
- Tissue damage
- Envenomation
- Infection by microorganisms (viruses, bacteria, malaria, Lyme)

Things That Bite:

The Golden Rules of Marine Bites: Sharks, Moray Eels, Sea Snakes, Barracuda, Squids, Seals

A – ASAP: Get the patient out of the water ASAP.

A – AIRWAY: Airway, Airway, Airway – monitor and manage.

B – BREATHING: Be prepared to provide artificial respirations as needed.

B – BLEEDING: Stop the BLEEDING with direct pressure.

In shark bite cases, it may be better to keep a wetsuit in place as this will help to apply direct pressure to the wounds.

C – CLEAN: Clean the wounds aggressively

D – DON'T: Do not suture or tightly close the wounds.

E – ENVIRONMENT: Get the patient dry and protect them from the environment; treat for shock as appropriate.

E – EVACUATE

Special Considerations:

If it is a Blue-ringed Octopus envenomation:

- Please remember this is a conscious paralysis.
- There is no available antivenom for the Blue-ringed Octopus.
- Transport ASAP for advanced care and respiratory support.

If it is a Sea Snake envenomation:

- Try to identify the snake.
- Apply a pressure immobilization splint to the bite site and involved extremity.
- Transport/Evacuate ASAP as they may require antivenom administration.

Long-term care:

- Monitor for and treat anaphylaxis.
- Monitor for infections.
- Consider tetanus prophylaxis.

Things That Stab:

Golden Rules If Stabbed, Impaled, or Harpooned: *Stingrays, Starfish, Sea Urchins, Lionfish, Rockfish, Stonefish, Stargazers, cone Shells*

A – ASAP: Get the patient out of the water ASAP.

A – AIRWAY: Airway, Airway, Airway – monitor and manage.

B – BREATHING: Be prepared to provide artificial respirations as needed.

B – BLEEDING: Stop the BLEEDING with direct pressure.

C – CONE SHELL: Consider whether they are going to require Cone Shell antivenoms.

D – DEBRIDE: Remove any spines, thorns, barbs, or harpoons and associated sheaths.

D – DUNK: Soak the affected area in non-scalding hot water for 60 – 90 minutes.

E – EVACUATE: Evacuate to definitive care ASAP.

Monitor for anaphylaxis.

Long-term care:

- Retained impaled objects are very common.
- Will require an x-ray to look for retained foreign body or spines.
- Secondary infections are very common.
- Consider tetanus prophylaxis.

Things That Sting:

Golden Rule for Things that Sting: *Jelly Fish, Sea Anemonies, Fire Corals*

A – ASAP: Get the patient out of the water ASAP.

A – AIRWAY: Airway, Airway, Airway – monitor and manage.

B – BREATHING: Be prepared to provide artificial respirations as needed.

B – BATHE: Neutralize the venom of the nematocyst with vinegar, alcohol, or urine.

Do not rinse with fresh water.

Remove the nematocyst with sand, scraping, or tape.

Avoid getting the nematocyst on anyone else.

Evacuate ASAP, and consider the use of antivenoms if appropriate.

MAMMALS

Despite the unlikelihood of being bitten by a wild animal, there are some general things to remember that may help prevent a bite from occurring:

- Never attempt to approach or feed a wild animal; they're called wild for a reason.
- Never throw food or food-waste overboard. Never attempt to feed animals like harbor-seals, which might appear tame but are still wild animals.
- Never tease or make aggressive movements toward wild animals.
- Bites may cause wounds: punctures, lacerations, avulsions.

Treatment:

- Stop the bleeding.
- Scrub the wound aggressively; try to move saliva out and away from the wound.
- Irrigate the wound generously with a dilute (1%) iodine solution.
- Do not close any animal bite in the field; the chance of infection is high.
- Is there a risk of rabies exposure? If so, consider rabies vaccine.

Although not all of these may a problem on the water, once you go ashore, you need this information.

SNAKES

- The primary reason people are bitten by snakes is that they pick them up.
- Bites usually occur on the hand.

Poisonous snakes of North America:

- Pit Vipers: They inject a hemotoxin that is meant to both poison and digest prey.
  - Rattlesnakes
  - Copperheads
  - Water Moccasins
- Coral Snake: Small, shy, and timid, this snake has a very powerful neurotoxin; however, bites are rare, and deaths are rarer.

Treatment of snake bites:

- Keep patient CALM.
- Monitor for anaphylaxis.
- Protect yourself and the scene; try to identify the snake, but don't risk a bite.
- Apply lymphatic compression wrap with 6" ACE wrap, distal to proximal and then proximal to distal; leave in place for the evacuation. Monitor pulses.
- Treat the wound and immobilize the extremity.
- Evacuate by carry-out or ambulation as appropriate.

INSECTS

◾ Hymenoptera: Bees, Hornets, Wasps, Fire Ants

Signs and Symptoms:

◾ Pain, local swelling, redness, and itching are common.

Treatment:

◾ Remove stinger/poison sack by scraping; do not use tweezers.

◾ Assess and Monitor for anaphylaxis.

◾ Use topical "bite and sting" stick for comfort.

◾ Give an oral antihistamine to prevent an allergic reaction: Benadryl (diphenhydramine) 25mg, 2 every
4 hours x 24 hours.

Ticks:

They are tiny septic tanks and carry several infectious diseases.

◾ Can spread Lyme Disease (the most common, but ticks can carry eight other diseases).

◾ Small to tiny with large abdomens and short legs.

◾ Color ranges from tan to brown, almost black.

◾ They attach to the host, bury their head in the skin, and take a blood meal for a day or more.

◾ Disease is spread by their saliva, an anticoagulant.

Treatment:

◾ Remove by pulling off (grasp as close to skin as possible); clean area well.

Mosquitoes and other blood-sucking insects:

◾ Can be vectors for infectious diseases: Malaria, Equine Enchephalitis, Nile Virus, etc.

◾ Avoid being bitten by using insect repellents, protective clothing, and sleeping under mosquito netting.

LIGHTNING

Laws of Nature:

- Lightning can and will do anything. It is unpredictable and uncontrollable.
- Lightning is most likely to strike the highest object around and follow the path of least resistance.

Rules to Live by:

- Thunderstorms are most dangerous as they approach, especially when within 1 mile.
- Don't be the highest object around to avoid a DIRECT STRIKE.
- Stay away from the highest objects to avoid SPLASH or STEP VOLTAGE.
- If on or near water, get off and away from the shoreline.
- Don't sit under overhangs or get into shallow caves.
- Lightning flows like water, so stay out of gullies and washes.
- Calculating Lightning's Distance—Light 286,000 miles/second vs. Sound 700 mph. Count the delay between flash and rumble: 5 seconds = 1 mile.
- Thunderstorms travel at approximately 20-25 mph, e.g. a storm approaching from 3 miles away (15 sec) will be in striking range in 6 minutes.
- Learn to "read a sky", monitor weather forcasts and warnings, and if you have warning and you have the option— get off the water

Places to Avoid or Get off:

- Ridges and cliff tops.
- Overhangs and shallow caves.
- Ditches, gullies, streams.
- Tall trees, poles, masts, high objects.
- Open areas, fields, meadows, any place in which you are the highest object.

What to Do If Caught Out:

 Get off the water if possible.

 Once off the water, seek out a low, dry spot among small trees.

 Stay away from tall trees, masts, cliff faces, and streams.

 Stay low in the boat–don't dangle a hand or foot in the water.

 CPR can be life-saving if initiated immediately, after victim has been struck by lightning.

Injuries: May Include:

- Respiratory arrest that can progress to cardiac arrest.
- Burns.
- Soft Tissue Injuries.
- Musculoskeletal injuries.

Treatment:

✓ Maintain ABCs; closely monitor for respiratory arrest.

✓ Do a complete physical exam.

✓ Treat all injuries.

✓ If conscious, force fluids to help prevent late complications.

✓ Evacuate.

GOOD POSITION: BELOW TREELINE, ON A PAD, NOT IN AREAS OF HIGHEST RISK.

SOLO

DIRECT STRIKE

TREELINE

LIGHTNING SPLASH

STEP VOLTAGE

DANGER AREA
1 MILE IN FRONT OF STORM

1 MILE

TREE LINE

LIGHTNING SPLASH
THE MOUTH OF A SHALLOW CAVE IS DANGEROUS!
STEP VOLTAGE

STREAM

LIGHTNING STRIKES:
- DIRECT STRIKE = WHEN YOU ARE THE OBJECT STRUCK. DON'T BE THE HIGHEST OBJECT.
- LIGHTNING SPLASH = WHEN SOMETHING NEAR YOU TAKES A DIRECT STRIKE & YOU GET SPLASHED. DON'T BE NEAR THE HIGHEST OBJECT.
- STEP VOLTAGE STRIKE = WHEN YOU ARE IN THE PATH OF LIGHTNING FLOW (VOLTAGE FLOWS LIKE WATER) & YOU BECOME A CONDUCTOR. STAY OUT OF SHALLOW CAVES, GULLIES, DITCHES, & STREAMS.

WATER = DANGER. ON A POND OR LAKE OR SEA YOU ARE THE HIGHEST POINT.

DATA COLLECTED BY: I. M. CONDUCTOR & I. B. STRUCK
TBRW

SURVIVAL ESSENTIALS:

ATTITUDE: THINK POSITIVELY.
- Positive attitude: belief that you can always make things better.
- Will to survive.

FOOD: GET FUEL TO BURN.
- High carbohydrate foods that require no preparation & provide quick energy.
- High carbohydrate foods that can be made into a warm drink (Jello).

WATER: QUENCH YOUR THIRST.
- Minimum of 2 liters per day if not active (up to 1-3 liters/hour if active).
- The ability to disinfect water (chemicals, filtering, boiling).

CLOTHING: STAY WARM & DRY.

- Warm clothing that retains heat even when wet (spare socks & hat).
- Waterproof rain gear, both tops and bottoms (large garbage or leaf bags).

SHELTER: GET DRY & STAY DRY.
- Is there a place on your boat that can be used to get out of the weather? If you can get ashore, do you have the ability to improvise a shelter?.
- Comfort & light (plumber's candles).

FIRE: GET WARM.
- Ability to build a fire—ashore—or a way to safely produce heat on board your boat.
- Ability to make kindling (pocket knife).
- Ability to warm water (tin cup).

NAVIGATION: KNOW WHERE YOU'RE GOING.

- Map & Compass; know how to use them.
- Ability to find your way at night (route-finding skills and flashlight and/or working navigation lights aboard a vessel).
- Ability to give your position on the radio.

WEATHER: KNOW THE ENVIRONMENT.

- Basic understanding of weather patterns.
- Knowledge of how to react to severe weather, lightning, etc.

SIGNALING: GET HELP.

- Whistle (preferably plastic) and signal mirror (whistle and/or mirror).
- VHF Radio. Know how to make a Mayday call or Pan Pan call.
- Know how to use signal flares, signal flags, or day shapes.

EXPERIENCE: PRACTICE SURVIVAL SKILLS BEFORE YOU NEED THEM.

- The most valuable and versatile survival tool is between your ears.

AVOID THE SURVIVAL SITUATION:

 Make a plan and work the plan.

 Know your limitations and the group's limitations.

SURVIVAL SKILLS:

Survival at Sea, or if marooned:
CRISIS INTERVENTION:

- Be prepared to heave to, or bivouac on a shore or island.

- Keep everyone warm and dry.

- Know how to use a VHF radio and how to contact the Coast Guard.

- Be able to radio a SOAP note.

- When calling for help:
  - Communicate your group's ability to stay put, or heave to.
  - Be sure you can give your position in either Latitude and Longitude or using known landmarks.
  - Know how to build a fire on land and make yourself very big, easy to find (surveyor's tape, Emergency flares, dye markers, streamers, or smoke flares, strobe light).

Factors that contribute to a crisis:

- Fatigue, taking on too much.

- Pushing hard or rushing to get someplace.

- Weather.

- Equipment failure or, more often, the wrong equipment.

- Lack of equipment.

- Personality problems.

- Poor judgment, making wrong decisions for wrong reasons—ego.

IF YOU WANT TO BE FOUND:

 Stay with the boat...

 Make yourself big and obvious:

- Rescue flares, distress signals, smoke flares, dye markers.
- Emergengy strobe light.
- Orange distress flag

THE ESSENTIALS FOR YOUR DITCH-BAG OR READY BAG:

- Spare hat—balaclava; can cover your whole face and neck.
- Spare socks—for feet and can also act as emergency mittens.
- Space blanket or big garbage/leaf bag.
- Metal cup—that you can hold over a candle or fire.
- JELL-O—with real sugar.
- Hard candies—with real sugar.
- Plumber's candles—short, thick, and long-burning.
- Waterproof matches—some people like to also carry a lighter.
- Compass.
- Plastic whistle and/or signaling mirror.
- Knife.
- Parachute cord—100".
- Stobe light-check and replace batteries regularly.
- Fluorescent dye packet.
- Chem light.
- Duct tape.
- Fresh water in packets or water bottle.
- Small med kit.

IF YOUR VESSEL IS OF SUFFICIENT SIZE:

- you should have a life raft, with "ditch bag" or "ready bag" easily accessible in an emergency situation, and survival suits if appropriate. PFDs (Life jackets) should be worn or readily available at all times.
- Personal Locator Beacons (PLB)have come down in price to under $300. You might want to consider having one in your ditch bag depending on the size of the vessel and how far off shore you are going to venture.

DITCH-BAGS FOR LARGER VESSELS MIGHT ALSO INCLUDE:

- Emergency Position-Indicating Radio Beacon, most commonly abbreviated as ***EPIRB***.
- Hand-held VHF radio.

SEASICKNESS

PROPRIOCEPTORS:

Throughout the body, especially located along the back and at the major joints, are specialized nerves called proprioceptors, or position sensors, that tell us where we are in space.

It is the combination of data streaming in from the eyes, ears, and proprioceptors that keep us oriented, upright, and balanced. This combination is what allows us to walk across a balance beam or tightrope, play sports, or even drive a car. Of the three the ears have the greatest input and control, and it is the ears that can cause the most trouble.

Motion sickness and seasickness, in particular, occur when all these neural signals flooding into the brain do not match up. When a mismatch has occurred, and the brain cannot properly interpret the data, vertigo, dizziness, and nausea are the result.

Symptoms of Seasickness:

- Early signs: yawning, sighing, and drowsiness that progress to:
- Dizziness
- Vertigo
- Headache
- Cold sweats
- Nausea
- Dry heaves
- Belching
- Vomiting (Usually, vomiting will relieve the nausea, at least temporarily. But, in the case of seasickness, vomiting does not.)

Treatment of Seasickness:

Treatment focuses on stabilizing the vestibular apparatus in the ears and shutting down the vomit or emetic center in the brain within the lateral reticular formation of the brainstem.

At the first warning signs of seasickness:

- Take the helm and steer if possible. Focus on and watch the distant horizon.
- If not steering, position yourself by getting to the midship or wheelhouse and ride the waves.
- Actively use your legs like pistons to keep your head and upper body as still as possible.
- Absorb the motion with your legs, as if you were skiing or skate boarding.
- If symptoms worsen, try to lie down in a well-ventilated area, flat on your back facing up, eyes closed, head still.

Drugs that can help seasickness:

Meclizine (Antivert, Bonine) 12.5 – 25mg by mouth every 6 hours as needed.

Dimenhydrinate (Dramamine) 50mg by mouth every 6 hours as needed.

Cinnarizine (Stugeron) 15mg by mouth every 6 hours as needed.

Scopolamine (Transderm-Scop) 1.5mg patch behind the ear which will last for 72 hours.

Scopolamine (Scopace) 0.4mg, 1 – 2 tabs by mouth every 8 hours as needed.

Promethazine (Phenergan) 12.5-25mg by mouth or by rectal suppository every 6 hours as needed. The suppository is especially useful for someone who is nauseous or vomiting.

Phenergan plus ephedrine (The "Coast Guard Cocktail") 25mg of each by mouth every 6 hours as needed.

DROWNING AND NEAR DROWNING

"Drowning is a process resulting in primary respiratory impairment from submersion in a liquid medium."

Definition agreed upon at the 2000 World Congress on Drowning.

pathophysiology of drowning

The pathophysiology of drowning is straightforward. The target organ is the lungs, and the cause of death is the resulting hypoxemia and acidosis.

The initial reactions to drowning include possible gasping for air, aspiration of water, or voluntary apnea (breath holding). Eventually, the hypoxemia leads to involuntary breathing and inhalation of water causing laryngospasm and rapid loss of consciousness. The apnea quickly leads to hypoxemia and acidosis, bringing on:

- Myocardial dysfunction
- Electrical instability and dysrythmias
- Eventual cardiac arrest
- CNS ischemia
- Asphyxiation and hypoxemia contribute to relaxation of the airway that allows water to enter the lungs ("wet drowning").
- During cardiac arrest, the muscles of the larynx relax also allowing water to enter the lungs.

Principles of Emergency Care of the Drowning Victim

You must get the victim to safety as quickly as possible, but, if they are struggling, they may pull you in with them—do not become a second victim.

Reach, Throw, Row, Go

Reach —extend your reach by using something long and rigid that the victim can grasp.

Throw —throw a rope, or something they can grasp to help stay afloat, and pull them to shore.

Row —get in a boat and row out to them. Do not try to get them into the boat; instead have them hang onto the boat and row them back to shore.

Go —the last option is for you to swim out to them, try to give them something to grasp, and tow them back to safety. Remember, if you decide to grab them and swim them back to shore, a victim who is panicking may overwhelm you and drown you as well! Do not attempt to rescue a struggling victim if you do not have training in water rescue. This training is readily available through the Red Cross.

Once the patient is safe

- Give primary attention to ABCs.
- Suspect spinal injury based on the mechanism of injury (MOI).
- If possible, take appropriate spinal cord injury precautions.
- If you perform CPR, you should anticipate vomiting, as the victim's stomach is usually full of water.
- Ensure the victim does not aspirate vomitus.
- Follow up—there is a risk of aspiration and delayed drowning or pneumonia.

Fresh vs. Salt

The controversy of drowning in salt versus fresh water has to do with osmosis. Water is drawn in the direction of higher salt concentration. If there is fresh water in the alveoli of the lungs, the water will rapidly move out of the alveoli and into the capillary vasculature surrounding the alveoli because there is more salt in the blood than in the fresh water. If there is salt water in the lungs, the higher salt concentration in the alveoli will draw water out of the pulmonary capillaries and into the alveoli. Both scenarios will also cause the surfactant lining of the alveoli to be rinsed or washed out of the lungs. Surfactant is a detergent-like compound that is essential to breathing because it has a unique property that helps to push and hold open the alveoli. Without it, when we exhale and the alveoli shrink in size, they will stick together like two sheets of glass with a thin film of water between them, making it much harder to inhale and fill the alveoli with fresh air. The result of drowning in fresh water versus salt water is the same, and it does not affect the emergency care skills needed to manage and resuscitate these patients.

— NOTES—

CHAPTER FOUR

SOFT TISSUE INJURIES
&
MEDICAL EMERGENCIES
From Minor Wounds to Critical Care

SOFT TISSUE INJURIES:

SOFT TISSUES:

- Everything except the bones.
- This section concentrates on insults and injuries to the skin and structures immediately under the skin: fat, muscles, & blood vessels.

Remember: Total Body Fluid Precautions—BSI

THE PIPES: ARTERIES, VEINS, & CAPILLARIES

They are muscular tubes that expand and contract depending on required blood flow.

- Arteries are the blood vessels leaving the heart.
    - They are under pressure: the systolic blood pressure—100 to 120 mmHg
    - Arteries are deep, protected, lying under the muscles directly on top of the bones.
    - When arteries are cut, they spurt like little oil wells—this is very rare.
- Veins are the blood vessels returning to the heart.
    - They are under very little pressure—10 to 20 mmHg pressure.
    - Veins are superficial and can be seen and felt under the skin.
    - When veins are cut, they drain blood. How much depends on the diameter of the vein.
- Capillaries are the tiny blood vessels that carry oxygen to the cells.
    - They are microscopic.
    - They are the most abundant vessels in the body.
    - One pound of body tissue has 1 mile of capillaries.
    - Capillaries in the skin expand and contract to control blood flow to the skin.
    - When cut, they seep or ooze blood

THE LIQUID: BLOOD—"THE RED STUFF"

- Carries oxygen, nutrients, and water to all the cells of the body.
- Carries away carbon dioxide and waste products.
- Carries heat into the extremities.
- Loss of blood causes a potentially life-threatening condition—SHOCK.

PRINCIPLES OF MANAGING SOFT TISSUE INJURIES:

- Control Bleeding
- Clean
- Bandage
- Monitor

TO CONTROL BLEEDING:

✔ Direct Pressure:
- Apply pressure directly over the wound and compress to stop the bleeding.
- Maintain pressure for about 10 minutes.

✔ Elevation:
- Along with direct pressure you can elevate the wound above the heart to decrease the pressure in the vessel, making it easier to stop the bleeding.

✔ Pressure Dressing:
- To maintain constant pressure, place something bulky and absorbent over the wound, an inch or two thick.
- Wrap the dressing with an elastic bandage for about 10 minutes.
- Then loosen the dressing to ensure circulation distal to the injury.
- Once bleeding has been controlled for 20–30 minutes, direct pressure can be stopped so the wound can be inspected and properly cleaned.

BUT WHAT IF...

✔ If unable to control bleeding with direct pressure and elevation:
- Remove the dressings and inspect the wound—you will find a spurting artery.
- Apply digital pressure with a finger to the little bleeder and hold pressure for ten minutes. (BSI!)

SPECIFIC SOFT TISSUE INJURIES:

Contusions:

■ Bruises: mild swelling, discoloration, may be painful.

✔ Rest, Ice, Compression, and Elevation (RICE) to limit swelling.

✔ Protect and watch injury closely in cold weather as it will freeze quicker than usual.

Abrasions:

■ Scrapes may be painful, dirty, and can easily become infected.

✔ Very little bleeding; while wound is pain-free, scrub thoroughly with soap & water.

✔ Allow to air dry before bandaging.

✔ You may apply antibiotic ointment for comfort.

Lacerations/Incisions:

■ May bleed profusely or require pressure dressing.

✔ Control bleeding and maintain hemostasis for 20–30 minutes.

✔ Cleanse well with copious irrigation.

✔ For large gaping wound—control bleeding, cleanse, approximate edges, don't close tightly.

🚫✔ If stitched or butterflied closed, infection is likely. It may have to be re-opened.

Flap Avulsion:

■ Three-sided tear, one side still attached.

✔ Control bleeding; then rinse under flap with water, and bandage it in its anatomical position.

Amputation:

- A body part is completely severed.

  - ✓ Wrap the part in a moist sterile dressing, and seal it in a plastic bag.

  - ✓ Immerse the bag in ice water, and evacuate both the patient and the part to the hospital.

Punctures:

- Small penetrating wound to the skin.

  - ✓ Gently irritate to cause some bleeding to flush out the wound.

  - ✓ Monitor for infection; this is the wound most likely to become infected.

Impaled Objects:

- Something stuck in the body that doesn't belong there.

  - ✓ Use common sense; if easily removed, remove it.

  - ✓ Once removed, use direct pressure to control bleeding..

- Impaled object may be removed if:

  - ✓ It is in an extremity.

  - ✓ It is in the cheek of the face (or buttocks).

  - ✓ It is metal in a cold environment.

  - ✓ It is too large or hard to cut off.

- Do not remove impaled objects if: (These objects should be bandaged in place.)
  - In the skull or neck.
  - In the chest, possibly into the lungs.
  - In the abdomen, possibly penetrating.

- What about fish hooks?

  - ✓ Easily removed by pushing away from the barb and backing out.

SOFT TISSUE INJURIES:

LONG-TERM WOUND CARE—DEFINITIVE CARE IS LONGER THAN 24 HOURS AWAY:

Prevent infection and promote healing by:

▪ Properly cleaning the wound—once bleeding has been controlled for 20-30 minutes:

✔ Remove dressings and closely inspect the wound.

✔ Check circulation, sensation, and motion (CSM) distal to the injury.

✔ Debride, remove any foreign material in the wound like sticks, grass, etc.

✔ Clean around the wound with soap & water or with a dilute solution of iodine.

✔ Clean the wound by irrigation with a forceful flow of sterile water or a dilute solution of iodine by using an irrigation syringe or water bottle.

✔ Cover the wound with dry sterile dressings and keep clean & dry.

✔ Bandage the sterile dressings in place.

✔ Change the dressings every 12 hours, and examine the wound for signs of infection.

But what if...

▪ If the wound is dirty or unable to be kept clean and dry:

✔ Cover the wound with a dressing soaked with a dilute solution of iodine, less than 2% strength.

✔ Change every 6 hours.

▪ There is impaired CSM distal to the injury:

✔ Do all of the above.

✔ Then splint.

✔ Then evacuate.

WOUND CARE DO'S AND DON'TS:

DO'S

 Protect from further injury, freezing, and from contamination by proper bandaging.

DON'TS

 Don't tightly close a wound with butterfly bandages or suturing.

 Don't fill the wound with an antibiotic ointment.

 Don't leave a pressure dressing in place for more than 20 minutes.

 Don't use tourniquets.

 Don't allow the wound to freeze.

 Don't be afraid of causing pain to properly clean a wound.

INFECTIONS:

- Caused by contamination of the wound by bacteria.
- Bacteria want to be warm, moist, and in the dark.
- Bacteria double (reproduce) every 30 minutes at 98°F (37°C).
- Signs and symptoms of an infection are a result of your immune system's response to the invading bacteria.
- Risk of tetanus; know shot status (good for ten years).

FECUNDITY GONE AWRY		
No. of Bacteria	*Elapsed Hours*	
1	*0*	*—*
16	*2*	*tens*
256	*4*	*hundreds*
1,024	*5*	*thousands*
131,072	*8.5*	*hundreds of thousands*
1,048,376	*10*	*millions*
1,073,537,024	*15*	*billions*
1,024,000,000,000	*20*	*trillions*
256,000,000,000,000	*24*	*256 trillion hungry little mouths to feed*

Signs of infection:

Early: localized to the skin and wound area:

- Red (rubor)—due to dilated capillary beds, increased blood flow to the area.
- Warm (calor)—due to the increased blood flow.
- Swollen (tumor)—due to the increased blood flow.
- Tender (dolor)—due to swelling.

Late—severe potentially life-threatening:

- Pus formation—collection of white blood cells, may be draining from the wound.
- Streaking up the extremity—due to infection traveling up lymphatics.
- Swollen and tender lymph nodes—the infection has reached the lymph nodes.
- Fever and Chills—a sign that the infection is spreading systemically, septic shock.

Treatment of skin infections:

- ✓ Apply moist heat packs; if possible, soak in hot water with salt.

- ✓ If the wound is closed but swollen, gently open so it can drain.

- ✓ Evacuate as soon as possible if red streaks and/or fever develop.

WHEN SHOULD YOU EVACUATE FOR STITCHES?

- If the cut goes through the skin (causes gaping) and is longer than 1 inch—cosmetic repair.
- If the cut is in the face, hands, or over a joint.
- If there is an injury to a nerve, ligament, or tendon.
- Check for distal CIRCULATION, SENSATION, and MOTION.

Burns

There are any number of possible ways to get a heat burn on a boat.

- Routine maintenance on a hot motor can result in a burn caused by flesh coming in contact with hot engine parts.
- Cooking on board a vessel poses a significant risk of getting burned because the galley is in motion.
- Spilled cooking fuel, the unhappy combination of electrical wiring and salt water, oil lamps. propane stored in ferrous metal containers, can all be situations that can lead to a fire on board a vessel.

Prevention

- Remember that simple tasks like cooking are potentially more dangerous on a boat, or while camping from a boat, than are those same tasks at home.
- Fire extinguishers can mean the difference between a minor fire with minimal damage, and major damage with burn victims. Be sure you have enough fire extinguishers on board, and make sure you know how to use them. Make sure everyone else on board knows how to use them. Remember US Coast Guard requirements are minimums.
- Be extra careful while handling flammable fluids like engine fuel, stove fuel, or lamp oil.

Treatment

THERMAL BURNS

Treatment: get the heat out:

✔ Remove clothing over and around the burn site.

✔ Cool with cold water for at least 15 minutes.

Superficial: First & Second Degree Burns:

- Appearance: area of the burn will turn red and may form blisters, but the patient has full sensation.

✔ Cold soak the burn with water for 15 minutes.

✔ Protect with a moist sterile dressing.

✔ Evacuate if the burn area is more than the size of their palm.

✔ If the burn area is large and painful, cover with moist dressings for comfort during evacuation.

Deep: Third Degree

Appearance: area of the burn may be red, white, charred, blistered, but there is no sensation; the burn is deep enough to destroy the sensory nerves.

 All deep burns must be evacuated.

Cold soak the burn with water for 15 minutes.

Cover with a moist dressing and waterproof bandage to prevent evaporation.

Hydrate—force fluids as burns can cause severe dehydration.

Chemical Burns

Many boats have starter batteries that contain acid. It is possible that in a collision, grounding, or knockdown, people on board can be exposed to the acid from a damaged battery resulting in chemical burns.

Prevention

The United States Coast Guard Auxiliary list of most common reasons that vessels fail a safety inspection includes unsecured batteries or improperly installed batteries in the top seven reasons that vessels fail voluntary safety inspections.

Most chemical burns are preventable though proper maintenance and following USCG approved safety guidelines.

Treatment

Remember scene safety—don't get any acid on yourself.

Stop the burn: remove the acid.

Rinse the burn with fresh water and baking powder to neutralize the acid.

Rope Burns

Rope burns are a combination injury; heat caused by friction often accompanied by an abrasion.

Prevention

- Seamanship. Know how to properly handle lines so that you don't get a rope burn.
- If you are handling lines that are going to run through your hands, wear sailing gloves.

Treatment

- Treat rope burns as heat burns.

- Treat any abrasions resulting from the injury as well.

Sunburns

Sunburn is typically just a nuisance that causes minor pain and a lost night's sleep. With proper care, the condition quickly resolves and a tan evolves. But, sunburn damage is permanent and cumulative. Repeated sunburns or chronic tanning increases aging effects on the skin producing wrinkles, areas of pigmentation, increased thickening, and precancerous skin lesions. (They are called precancerous because with time they will become cancers—basal cell cancer, squamous cell cancer, or malignant melanoma

Prevention

- All sunburns are preventable by using proper clothing, hats, umbrellas (bumbershoots), sunblock, and even avoiding the sun.

Treatment

- Assess for signs of heat exhaustion and heat stroke.
- Hydrate with a water and salt replacement solution to prevent dehydration.
- Pain and discomfort are well-controlled with non-steroidal anti-inflammatory drugs (NSAID) such as ibuprofen (Advil, Motrin) or naprosyn (Aleve). Acetaminophen (Tylenol) is not an NSAID, but, it does work well to relieve pain and can be taken with a NSAID for added pain control.
- Moisturize the skin with a good skin cream that contains aloe.
- Stay out of the sun and wear sunblock or cover up with clothing to prevent further skin damage.
- If blisters occur, leave them intact.
- Be aware that certain medications do cause photosensitivity to UV light and, therefore, increase the likelihood and severity of a sunburn. If you are taking a photosensitizing drug, it is very important to wear a proper sunblock.

BLISTERS:

- Caused by friction against the skin forcing the layers of the skin apart.
- Common causes are a loose boot or shoe rubbing against the heel, or a shovel handle or oar-loom rubbing against the palms of the hands.
- The body reacts to the abuse by secreting water into the area of trauma.
- Blisters start out as a "hot spot" that, if left unattended to, will grow into a water-filled blister or bleb.

Treatment:

- React to the pain or "hot spot."

  - ✔ If on the foot, remove the sock and boot and apply athletic tape over the hot spot.

  - ✔ Then redress the foot paying attention to how the sock and boot fit.

- If a fluid-filled blister has formed, properly treat and protect the blister.

  - ✔ Clean the area around the blister.

  - ✔ Drain the blister by making small holes around the base with a sterile needle, and gently compress the blister to force out the fluid.

  - ✔ Surround the blister with padding, moleskin, molefoam, Spenco Second Skin, etc.

  - ✔ Fill the well created by the blister dressing with an antibiotic ointment to protect the fragile skin and minimize friction.

  - ✔ Cover the blister area and padding with tape.

  - ✔ If on the foot, redress the foot.

  - ✔ Clean daily and monitor for signs of infection.

PREVENTION:

- Sock combination—thin on skin, thick over
- Properly fit boots
- React early to pain or hot spots
- Keep feet dry—wet feet blister easily and quickly

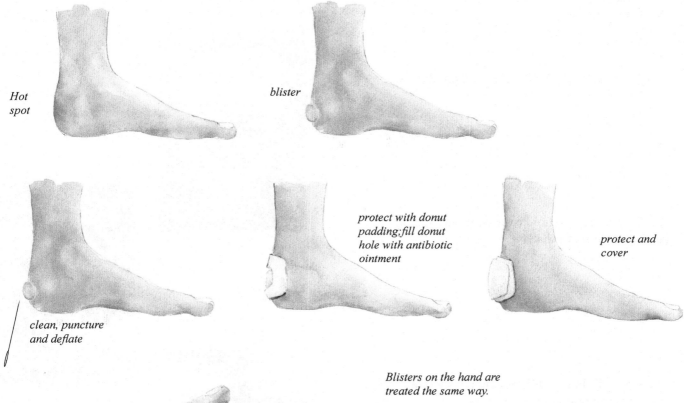

Hot spot

blister

clean, puncture and deflate

protect with donut padding; fill donut hole with antibiotic ointment

protect and cover

Blisters on the hand are treated the same way.

Part of prevention of blisters is keeping the area in question dry, this can be difficult to do when rowing and paddling.

SOFT TISSUE INJURIES:

BANDAGING SKILLS:

Dressing: Sterile material put directly onto a wound site.
- Sterile gauze pads: 2" x 2" or 4" x 4" trauma dressings.

Bandage: Piece of material that holds the dressings in place.
- Cravat: A large triangular piece of material that is used in very clever ways to hold dressings.
- ACE bandage: Elastic material 2" to 6" wide that can be used to hold dressings and also to apply compression.
- Roller gauze/ Kling: Soft, fluffy material in a roll, 1" to 6" wide that can be wrapped to hold a dressing in place.

Specific Bandages:

- **Scalp bandage**: To hold a dressing on the scalp.

- **Temporal/Jaw**: To hold a dressing on the side of the head, or to support the jaw.

- **Shoulder**: To hold a dressing on the shoulder or upper arm and maintain range of motion.

Arm sling & swathe: To support the shoulder, upper arm, elbow, forearm, or wrist.

Hip: To hold a dressing on the hip or buttocks and maintain full range of motion of the hip.

Knee: To hold a dressing on the knee and maintain full range of motion.

Sprained ankle: RICE
(If needed, use the ankle bandage shown in the Musculoskeletal chapter.)

MEDICAL EMERGENCIES & CRITICAL CARE:

These are rare but potentially life-threatening problems you need to be able to recognize and manage. A good history will usually make the diagnosis.

CHANGE IN LEVEL OF CONSCIOUSNESS:

Level of Consciousness (LOC) is maintained by the brain, so any change indicates a brain problem. **Signs and Symptoms:**

✔ Change in personality.

✔ Deteriorating LOC, **A** > **V** > **P** > **U** > **Death**

✔ Seizure activity.

Causes: Your brain needs four things to survive and thrive; causes of change in LOC:

✔ Oxygen (hypoxia).

✔ Carbohydrates (glucose, hypo/hyperglycemia).

✔ Proper temperature, 98.6^0F/37^0C (hypo/hyperthermia).

✔ Proper pressure = intracranial pressure (ICP).

Principles of Management

✔ Maintain and monitor the airway & breathing.

✔ Place in the Recovery Position to protect the airway.

✔ If respiratory rate less than 10 or greater than 30, assist breathing—1 breath every 5 seconds.

✔ Recognize the problem early and evacuate early as these problems tend to steadily deteriorate.

✔ If suspicious of a diabetic emergency, give them sugar.

✔ Get help; this patient needs to be evacuated ASAP.

SHORTNESS OF BREATH (SOB)—AIRWAY, BREATHING:

- The brain perceives that it is not getting enough oxygen so it causes a sensation of SOB.
- So, either there is not enough oxygen getting into the blood, or there is not enough oxygenated blood getting to the brain.

Signs and Symptoms:

- Complaining of shortness of breath.
- Rapid shallow or deep breathing.
- Skin color pale to cyanotic (blue) as hypoxia increases.
- May be wheezing.

Causes:

- Lungs: asthma (wheezing).
- Lungs: pneumothorax (no breath sounds on one side)
- Lungs: pulmonary edema, pneumonia (crackles).
- Lungs: pulmonary emboli (dyspnea).
- Heart: MI, angina (chest pain).
- Anaphylaxis, anxiety, altitude.

Principles of Management:

 Look: is your patient struggling to breathe—mouth open, obvious effort. Are they cyanotic; do they have hives?

 Listen to the breath sounds: is there wheezing, gurgling, or no breath sounds on one side?
- Support respirations; sitting up may help.
- Assist breathe for them if they cannot move enough air on their own.
- If asthmatic, may use **<u>THEIR</u>** rescue inhaler: Albuterol Metered Dose Inhaler (MDI), 2 puffs every 10 minutes until breathing improves (up to 4 times), then 2 puffs every 4 hours.

 If yes to these symptoms, get help—this patient needs to be evacuated **ASAP**.

ASTHMA

Allergens in the airway cause swelling, bronchospasm, and increased mucous production in the bronchioles. This causes the bronchioles to narrow resulting in wheezing, air trapping, and shortness of breath.

Signs and Symptoms:

- Shortness of breath.
- Word dyspnea—unable to count to ten on one breath.
- Expiratory wheezing—audible initially with auscultation.

Treatment:

- CALM the patient, and remain calm yourself.
- Place in position of comfort (usually sitting or semi-sitting).
- Take a good history—find out which medications, if any, have been taken.
- Assist with the use of rescue metered dose inhaler, Albuterol, or Xopenex.
- Encourage pursed-lip breathing to create backpressure and open bronchioles.
- May do lateral chest compressions to help remove trapped air.
- Consider evacuation.

CHEST PAIN:

- There are many harmless things that cause chest pain, such as indigestion, heartburn, pulled chest wall muscles.
- Your concern with chest pain is the chance that it is cardiac.

Signs and Symptoms (cardiac):

- Left-sided, substernal chest pain that may radiate into the left arm.
- Associated with a sensation of shortness of breath.
- Associated with a cold sweat.
- Is made worse by exertion and anxiety.

Causes:

- Non-cardiac: indigestion, heartburn, pulled muscles.
- Cardiac: acute MI, angina.

Principles of Management for Suspected Cardiac Pain:

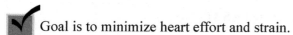

- Goal is to minimize heart effort and strain.

- Unless you are absolutely certain that the pain is not cardiac, evacuate.

- The cardiac patient should be kept at rest, as exertion will make the pain worse.

- Transport in a position of comfort to support breathing.

✔ Keep them calm, reassure.

✔ If you have aspirin with you, give them 1 adult or 4 baby aspirin (unless allergic to aspirin).

✔ Get help; this patient needs to be evacuated **ASAP**.

ANAPHYLACTIC REACTION:

▢ Is a severe, life-threatening allergic reaction.

Signs and Symptoms:

■ The patient usually knows if they are allergic and will tell you (but ask anyway).

■ They may have a rash—hives.

■ They may have increasing shortness of breath.

■ They may feel increasingly anxious, even terrified.

■ They may wheeze and/or have difficulty breathing or speaking.

Causes:

■ Bee stings (Hymenoptera: bees, wasps, hornets, fire ants).

■ Foods, especially peanuts or seafood.

■ Medications, e.g. penicillin.

Principles of Management:

✔ Immediately give antihistamine: Benadryl, 50mg every 4 hours for 24 hours; other antihistamines will also work.

✔ If they begin to lose their airway (SOB, wheezing), give epinephrine with an Epi-Pen or Twinject.

✔ Once able to breathe and swallow, give them the antihistamine as explained above.

✔ A second dose of epinephrine may be given if the first dose wears off before the antihistamine is absorbed.

✔ Evacuate immediately.

APPENDICES

SOLO—A LOOK AT WHO WE ARE

The 1970's

SOLO took root in the early 1970s and grew out of the vision of its founders Frank Hubbell and Lee Frizzell (husband and wife). As Frank recalls, pre-hospital care was in its infancy, and an organized EMS system didn't exist yet in New Hampshire. The concept of providing emergency care to the sick and injured revolved around what is today referred to as the "Golden Hour." "As skiers, climbers, and EMTs in the White Mountains of New Hampshire, we would respond to the call for injured hikers and climbers," Frank remembers. "It very quickly became apparent that the skills that we had learned as "street EMTs" did not work in the wilderness environment. We had to learn how to provide care outside the golden hour. But, that information was not available—we had to learn it through experience." Frank's frustration with the lack of an appropriate "wilderness" standard led to the creation of one of the first, if not the first, wilderness emergency medicine courses in the country. By 1975, a basic "Mountain/Woods First Aid" course was taken on the road by Frank, and taught to the few folks who could see its value. That course outline and objectives remain the foundation of our most popular course today, Wilderness First Aid. In 1976, Frank, and his wife Lee Frizzell, a trained educator, began growing the dream of creating a school to develop and teach various aspects and levels of outdoor/wilderness medicine. They named that school SOLO, for Stonehearth Open

SOLO's Main Building, Kaila Hall

Learning Opportunities. In the next year, 1977, Frank taught the first official SOLO course in his parents' living room. The same SOLO team soon broke ground on Tasker Hill, just south of Conway, and began construction of the unique three-story post-and-beam structure that would become SOLO's headquarters. Today this building houses our main classrooms and stands as the centerpiece of our expanding campus. While the Main Building (Kaila Hall) was being completed, another structure, the Octagon, was constructed as a kitchen and dining facility. The campus, although somewhat rustic, was now in full operation. Over the next two years, SOLO ran more than 30 courses for organizations like Outward Bound, the AMC, and numerous college and university outing clubs. Putting their new knowledge to the test, these groups found that SOLO offered the most valuable training in first aid they had ever been exposed to. Word of these amazing courses spread throughout the outdoor education industry, and by the end of the decade, SOLO had become a full-time passion and a full-time business.

The 1980's

In the next few years SOLO would develop the three-day EMT Refresher Training Program (1980) and the month-long Wilderness EMT program (1980) which both have become industry standards; and, in 1983, SOLO received full approval for its courses from both the State of New Hampshire Office of Emergency Medical Services and the National Registry of EMTs. In 1982, Frank had decided to further his medical education and entered Northeastern University's Physician Assistant program, becoming certified in 1984. Several significant events in the annals of wilderness medicine occurred in the mid 1980s. SOLO created the Wilderness First Responder program, which seemed a logical step after having designed the Wilderness EMT program, and collaborated with a newly formed organization, Wilderness Medical Associates (WMA) to offer this brand new course at an Outward Bound site. Two students in this first class soon joined the small SOLO staff and spent the next few years learning wilderness medicine and teaching SOLO programs around the country. Expressing a desire to establish a base in the West, they left with SOLO's blessing and established a base in Colorado to provide SOLO training to SOLO's already established western sponsors. Soon, this "SOLO West" venture became the Wilderness Medicine Institute (WMI). Until being acquired by the National Outdoor Leadership School (NOLS), WMI offered SOLO certifications.

During this time, SOLO founded the Wilderness Medicine Newsletter, and the staff published articles in that and other major EMS journals. Lee left her teaching career to take over the role of SOLO's director when Frank went off to the New England College of Osteopathic Medicine to become a physician. In 1988, SOLO staff helped develop wilderness medicine clinical guidelines through the American Society for Testing and Materials (ASTM) Wilderness Medical Task Group. These guidelines were later adopted by the National Association of EMS Physicians. At this same time, SOLO was featured in a Turner Broadcasting Systems program on New Hampshire. 1990 was another busy year, highlighted by publication of the first edition of Medicine for the Backcountry by Frank Hubbell and Buck Tilton.

SOLO founder Frank Hubbell teaching in 1980

The 1990's

As if all that wasn't enough, Frank graduated from medical school in 1991 with several academic awards and "Graduate with Distinction" honors. Shortly after graduation, Frank was appointed to a position on New Hampshire's Medical Control Board; a position he continues to hold today.

In the mid-90s, SOLO bought and rebuilt an apartment house adjacent to the campus. The revamped building became Toad Hall, a 30-person dormitory named from Kenneth Grahame's The Wind in the Willows. The school also began formal outdoor leadership training with the inaugural Advanced Leadership and Emergency Care (ALEC) class. Our reputation and popularity caught the attention of the PBS television series Trailside, which featured a segment filmed at the Tasker Hill campus. Accreditation from the University System of New Hampshire was sought in 1996, and a committee from the system reviewed SOLO programs and approved credits for students enrolled in the College of Lifelong Learning (now Granite State College). SOLO continued to be represented at important conferences, including those for the Association for Experiential Education, Northern New Hampshire EMS, the Wilderness Risk Managers, and many others. SOLO was accredited to offer continuing education through the Continuing Education Coordinating Board for

Emergency Medical Services (CECBEMS) for the Wilderness EMT Module. In 1998, SOLO was featured in the Encyclopedia Britannica's Health and Medicine supplement, and in 1999, we were the focus of a Time magazine column on Wilderness 911.

The New Millenium

The year 2000 saw SOLO's wilderness medical protocols reviewed and formally adopted by the State of NH and the awarding of undergraduate credit for many of SOLO's programs through Vermont's Sterling College. In addition, several schools joined the growing number of colleges offering SOLO programs on a semester basis. 2001 marked SOLO's official 25th anniversary and the undertaking of the development of the CARE program with the State of New Hampshire. Twelve, one-day seminars for fire, rescue, and law enforcement personnel were delivered by SOLO during 2002.

Throughout 2002, SOLO focused much energy on establishing TMC Books, and before the end of the year, their first publication, Merlin and the Black Star, was out. In early 2003, TMC published An Ice Climber's Guide to Northern New England soon to be followed by SOLO's Field Guide to Wilderness First Aid and Whitehorse Ledge Rock Climbing Topo Map. Several more colleges offered SOLO semester programs, and the number is still growing. Highlights of 2004, included SOLO's providing first aid training for the staff and crew of PBS's Colonial House; SOLO's WEMT course receiving licensure from the State of New Hampshire's Postsecondary School Commission; Frank Hubbell being the recipient of NH's prestigious David J. Connor EMS Appreciation Award in recognition of his long-term dedication to NH's Emergency Medical Services; and SOLO's being honored with the "Educator of the Year" award at the Northern New Hampshire's EMS Conference.

The release of TMC Books' lavishly illustrated book, Treehouse Chronicles, was a highpoint of 2005. The book was widely praised for its literary and artistic merit, was called one of the "Best Outdoor Books of 2005" by the chairman of the National Outdoor Book Awards, and went on to win five national book awards. The Wilderness Medicine Newsletter (WMN) continued to grow, both in size and distribution, as people responded to the new online format—which made the WMN available anywhere in the world at the click of a mouse. Before year's end, an exciting new set of courses was launched including T/E/A/M (Travel/Ecotourism/Adventure Travel/Medicine—now grouped under International Medicine), and a faith-based Missionary Medicine program. The January issue of Outside Magazine gave the nod to SOLO courses in an article entitled "50 Ways to Live Large" as one of the 50 things from around the world that you need to do before you die, and AMC Outdoors featured a piece on the SOLO WFR program in their November 2005 issue.

Repairs and renovations on the campus were our main focus throughout 2006. A new multi-function classroom, replacing the Kaila Hall deck, was the most noticeable project. TMC continued to garner awards for their book, Treehouse Chronicles, bringing the total to eight, and by the end of the year TMC had published the full set of NH State EMS Protocols.

One of the most exciting developments in recent SOLO history occurred in 2007 with the formalization of a partnership between Nantahala Outdoor Center, the premier whitewater facility in the US, and SOLO. NOC established a SOLO Southeast base with a separate office dedicated to SOLO Wilderness Medical courses. Like other SOLO centers which include San Juan EMS in the Northwest and CAMRA in the Southwest, NOC has helped continue SOLO's strong presence in the South as it develops new sponsors throughout the region. 2008 was a year of course growth and TMC's publication of Brian Walsh's "Boys Should Be Boys." SOLO was present at a number of regional and national conferences and entered into our second year of providing programs in several African countries. Also, Lee was honored with the Northern New Hampshire Emergency Medical Services Council's Leadership award acknowledging her 30 year of service in EMS education.

Planning the future in 2002

After many, many years of a leaky Main Building roof and many, many attempts to patch said roof, the summer of 2009, on record as one of the wettest in NH history, was the impetus that caused the roof to finally be replaced! The new roof, which, unfortunately, had to be constructed during a WEMT course, has proven to be watertight. We appreciated the students' forbearance with the project. Another major building project involved filling in the "pit," creating a continous surface on the first floor. More on that in another section. The big focus in 2010 has been SOLO's commitment to and ongoing work with Haitian relief with weekly teams going out and one instructor on the ground for almost 2 months coordinating efforts.

Thirty years after the official founding of SOLO, interest in wilderness medicine training is still growing. Eight, month-long WEMT courses are offered on our campus annually along with several dozen other programs. Since SOLO has been a licensed NH rescue unit for years, our staff and students continue to volunteer on backcountry search and rescue missions in the White Mountains. SOLO courses are increasingly offered in the West as new sites for ongoing SOLO training are being developed. Strategic partnerships with the San Juan Islands, WA, EMS, Central Arizona Mountain Rescue Association, Learn Outdoors, also in Arizona, Apex in Colorado, and Aspen Education Group have resulted in SOLO training being available on a regular basis. SOLO instructors can now be found in most western states. From a gathering in a living room over a quarter century ago, SOLO has grown into a large, diverse organization: a leader not only in medicine, but also in education and standards as well. From basic first aid—still the foundation of SOLO's purpose—we now find instructors teaching around the country as well as internationally, reaching outdoor users, trip leaders, expeditioners, disaster relief workers, missionaries, and physicians. By the end of 2006, over 110,000 people had taken a SOLO class.

Part I quiz: Response and Assessment   **Student Name** _____

1. Which of the following are common modes of transmission of infectious disease?
   - ☐ a. Airborne by inhaling infectious particles.
   - ☐ b. Vector or insect bite.
   - ☐ c. Waterborne by drinking contaminated water.
   - ☐ d. Direct contact or bloodborne.
   - ☐ e. All of the above.

2. The purpose of the Primary Survey is all of the following except:
   - ☐ a. Find and treat all potentially life-threatening problems.
   - ☐ b. Protect from the environment.
   - ☐ c. Prevent any further injury.
   - ☐ d. Establish and monitor vital signs.

3. The Secondary Survey consists of:
   - ☐ a. Vital signs.
   - ☐ b. Patient exam.
   - ☐ c. AMPLE history.
   - ☐ d. SOAPNOTE.
   - ☐ e. All of the above.

4. All of the following AMPLE history explanations are correct except for:
   - ☐ a. A = allergies.
   - ☐ b. M = medications.
   - ☐ c. P = previous injuries or illness.
   - ☐ d. L = last in and out.
   - ☐ e. E = environmental conditions.

5. The Objective part of the SOAPnote will contain all of the following except:
   - ☐ a. Heart rate, respiratory rate and effort, & level of consciousness.
   - ☐ b. Description of locations of pain, tenderness, and injuries.
   - ☐ c. AMPLE history.
   - ☐ d. Condition of the group as a whole.

6. The rescue plan consists of all of the following except:
   - ☐ a. The group's condition.
   - ☐ b. Treating the patient's injuries.
   - ☐ c. The group's level of preparedness.
   - ☐ d. Sending for help.

Part II quiz: Trauma: Musculoskeletal Injuries: **Student Name** _____

1. A sprain or strain can cause injury to all of the following except:
   - ☐ a. Muscle.
   - ☐ b. Tendon.
   - ☐ c. Ligament.
   - ☐ d. Bone.

2. All of the following are correct for treating a sprain except:
   - ☐ a. Rest, stop, and sit down.
   - ☐ b. Ice for vasoconstriction.
   - ☐ c. Compression with an ACE bandage.
   - ☐ d. Elevation to decrease circulation to the affected area.
   - ☐ e. Mild exercise to encourage healing.

3. Which of the following statements regarding fractures is correct?
   - ☐ a. There is typically point tenderness over the fracture site.
   - ☐ b. The patient may have felt something snap, crack, or pop.
   - ☐ c. There may be discoloration, swelling, or deformity.
   - ☐ d. There is a loss of normal function.
   - ☐ e. All are correct.

4. The most important aspect of fracture care is to:
   - ☐ a. Maintain normal function and range of motion.
   - ☐ b. Maintain circulation distal to the site of the injury.
   - ☐ c. Adjust the fracture site until there is normal sensation and movement.
   - ☐ d. Splint the fracture exactly the way you found it.

5. The reason to straighten out an angulated fracture is to:
   - ☐ a. Make it easier to splint.
   - ☐ b. Place the injury in a more comfortable position.
   - ☐ c. Establish and maintain circulation.
   - ☐ d. Place it in the proper position for healing.

6. Splints should be monitored every 15 minutes to:
   - ☐ a. Make sure that the splint is still tight and snug.
   - ☐ b. Make sure the fracture is in the proper position.
   - ☐ c. Make sure the extremity is staying cool so that it will not swell.
   - ☐ d. Make sure there is circulation distal to the fracture.

7. Which of the following statements is incorrect regarding spinal injuries?
   - ☐ a. The patient must by sober and oriented x 3 to "clear" the spine.
   - ☐ b. The patient should be free of distracting injuries at the time of the exam.
   - ☐ c. If they fell more than twice their height, you must treat for a back injury.
   - ☐ d. You can move the patient from position of injury to position of function.

Part III quiz: Environmental Emergencies   **Student Name** _____

1. Circle True or False in regard to the following statements about hypothermia:

    T / F   Hypothermia is most commonly associated with cold, wet, windy conditions.

    T / F   Humans are designed to lose heat when wet.

    T / F   Hypothermia has little or no effect on the human brain.

    T / F   Humans burn glucose as a fuel to help maintain body temperature.

    T / F   Shivering is involuntary muscular contractions that produce heat.

    T / F   Shivering does NOT impair other physical activity.

    T / F   Conscious hypothermia victims need water and glucose.

    T / F   Never expose and dry off a wet hypothermia patient.

2. Which of the following is incorrect regarding frostbite?

    ☐ a. Superficial frostbite can be field rewarmed with skin-to-skin contact.

    ☐ b. Deep frostbite should not be field rewarmed, but should be protected from further damage.

    ☐ c. Refreezing recently thawed frostbite will cause a much worse injury.

    ☐ d. It is preferable to use hot air to thaw frostbitten hands.

3. Which of the following is correct regarding heat stroke?

    ☐ a. Heat stroke is a minor injury associated with dehydration and salt depletion.

    ☐ b. Heat stroke is self-correcting and does not require treatment.

    ☐ c. Heat stroke patients need to be aggressively cooled with water.

    ☐ d. Heat stroke is rarely associated with dehydration.

4. When someone is sent out to get help, all of the following are true except:

    ☐ a. Keep everyone busy, and keep everyone warm and dry.

    ☐ b. Build a bivouac to protect the patient and everyone else in the group.

    ☐ c. Build a fire or light a stove to make something warm to drink.

    ☐ d. Send someone out for help every 1 – 2 hours until help arrives.

Part IV quiz: Soft Tissue Injuries and Critical Care   **Student Name** _____

1. All of the following statements are correct except:
   - ☐ a. Blood is sterile and harmless to others exposed to it.
   - ☐ b. Arteries are under pressure, and although rare, spurt blood when cut.
   - ☐ c. Veins are low pressure and drain blood when cut.
   - ☐ d. Capillaries are very small and low pressure; they ooze or seep when cut.
   - ☐ e. Veins are commonly injured because they can be just under the skin.

2. All of the following statements about controlling bleeding are correct except:
   - ☐ a. Pressure directly over the wound is the most effective way to control bleeding.
   - ☐ b. If direct pressure is not enough, you can also elevate the wound.
   - ☐ c. Pressure dressings are very effective but should only be used for about 10 minutes.
   - ☐ d. Never remove a dressing once it has been placed on the wound.
   - ☐ e. In extreme cases direct digital pressure can be applied directly to an open spurting artery.

3. All of the following are signs or symptoms of a localized tissue infection except:
   - ☐ a. The area is red (rubor).
   - ☐ b. The area is warm to the touch (calor).
   - ☐ c. The area is swollen (tumor).
   - ☐ d. The area is tender to the touch (dolor).
   - ☐ e. The area is red but not warm to the touch.

4. Please answer True or False about severe potentially life-threatening tissue infections:
   - T / F   There can be a collection of pus or other drainage coming from the wound.
   - T / F   There may be red streaks running proximally from the infection site.
   - T / F   There may be swollen tender lymph nodes proximal to the infection site.
   - T / F   The patient may have fever and chills.
   - T / F   Wound infections can be prevented by proper cleaning and bandaging.
   - T / F   It takes at least 3 days for a potentially life-threatening infection to occur.
   - T / F   Wounds associated with impairment of circulation, sensation, or movement
             do not need to be immediately evacuated; they can wait 2 – 3 days.

5. Which statement is incorrect in regard to impaled objects?
   - ☐ a. Never remove impaled objects.
   - ☐ b. Remove impaled objects that are in an extremity.
   - ☐ c. Remove metal impaled objects in a cold environment.
   - ☐ d. Do not remove impaled objects in the skull, neck, chest, or abdomen.

6. Which of the following statements is incorrect about thermal burns.
   - ☐ a. Immediately cold soak the burn area with cold water for about 15 minutes.
   - ☐ b. Superficial burns rarely cause very much pain.
   - ☐ c. Deep burns have minimal pain due to nerve destruction in the skin.
   - ☐ d. All deep burns patients need to be hydrated and evacuated.

SOAPNOTE

Subjective: age, sex, mechanism of injury (MOI), chief complaint(C/C): _____

_____

_____

_____

_____

Objective: vital signs, patient exam, AMPLE history:

Vital Signs

TIME					
LOC oriented x ?					
RR & effort					
HR & effort					
Skin C, T, M					

Patient Exam: Describe locations of pain, tenderness & injuries: _____

_____

_____

Allergies: _____

Medications:_____

Past pertinent medical history:_____

Last in and out:_____

Events leading up to accident:

_____

Assessment: problem list:

1._____

2._____

3._____

Plan: plan for each problem on the problem list:

1._____

2._____

3._____

4. MONITOR - How often do you plan to monitor the patient? _____

© 2007 SOLO

SOAPNOTE

Subjective: age, sex, mechanism of injury (MOI), chief complaint(C/C): _____

_____

_____

_____

_____

Objective: vital signs, patient exam, AMPLE history:

Vital Signs

TIME					
LOC oriented x ?					
RR & effort					
HR & effort					
Skin C, T, M					

Patient Exam: Describe locations of pain, tenderness & injuries: _____

_____

_____

Allergies: _____

Medications:_____

Past pertinent medical history:_____

Last in and out:_____

Events leading up to accident:

_____

Assessment: problem list:

1._____

2._____

3._____

Plan: plan for each problem on the problem list:

1._____

2._____

3. _____

4. MONITOR - How often do you plan to monitor the patient? _____

SOAPNOTE

Subjective: age, sex, mechanism of injury (MOI), chief complaint(C/C): _____

_____

_____

_____

_____

Objective: vital signs, patient exam, AMPLE history:

Vital Signs

TIME					
LOC oriented x ?					
RR & effort					
HR & effort					
Skin C, T, M					

Patient Exam: Describe locations of pain, tenderness & injuries: _____

_____

_____

Allergies: _____

Medications:_____

Past pertinent medical history:_____

Last in and out:_____

Events leading up to accident:

_____

Assessment: problem list:

1._____

2._____

3._____

Plan: plan for each problem on the problem list:

1._____

2._____

3. _____

4. MONITOR - How often do you plan to monitor the patient? _____

SOAPNOTE

Subjective: age, sex, mechanism of injury (MOI), chief complaint(C/C): _____

_____

_____

_____

_____

Objective: vital signs, patient exam, AMPLE history:

Vital Signs

TIME					
LOC oriented x ?					
RR & effort					
HR & effort					
Skin C, T, M					

Patient Exam: Describe locations of pain, tenderness & injuries: _____

_____

_____

Allergies:_____

Medications:_____

Past pertinent medical history:_____

Last in and out:_____

Events leading up to accident:

_____

Assessment: problem list:

1._____

2._____

3._____

Plan: plan for each problem on the problem list:

1._____

2._____

3. _____

4. MONITOR - How often do you plan to monitor the patient? _____

Certificate of Completion

This certificate is presented to

_____

For completion of the two-day course in

Wilderness First Aid Afloat

Instructors: _____

Dates: _____   Exp. _____

Resources

United States Coast Guard

US Coast Guard website www.uscg.mil

US Coast Guard Navigation Center—Navigation Center Local Notice to Mariners www.navcen.uscg.gov

US Coast Guard Boating Safety Resource Center www.uscgboating.org

US Coast Guard Auxiliary www.cgaux.org

Weather and Navigation

National Oceanic And Atmospheric Administration www.noaa.gov

GRIB weather forcast data www.grib.us/Home.aspx

NOAA Raster navigational charts www.nauticalcharts.noaa.gov/mcd/Raster/index.htm

Boater Safety and Seamanship

Boater Safety programs for 42 states www.boat-ed.com

National Association of State Boating Law Enforcement www.nasbla.org

Boat US www.boatus.com/

SOLO

We hope that you enjoy your SOLO course. SOLO is the nation's leader in wilderness medicine education with over 110,000 students attending courses since 1976. SOLO has been instrumental in the development of Wilderness First Aid, Wilderness First Responder, and Wilderness

EMT curricula. Our campus, perched on 300 acres in the heart of New Hampshire's White Mountains, is a unique teaching facility made up of our three-story Main Building, a 30-person dorm, dining hall, and other facilities. Find out more about SOLO by visiting www. soloschools.com. We hope you decide to continue your wilderness medicine education by attending one of our other programs. SOLO, PO Box 3150, Conway, NH 03818 • 603-447-6711

WMN *Wilderness Medicine Newsletter*

SOLO has produced the *Wilderness Medicine Newsletter* continuously since 1988. It is dedicated to disseminating information on medical issues and practices in the backcountry. The newsletter is a full-color online journal that comes out six times each year. Subscribers download each issue by signing onto the TMC Books website with a login and password. Because it is online, the newsletter is available anytime, anywhere in the world at the click of a mouse. A one year subcription is just $15. You can purchase a subscription to the newsletter online and get more information by visiting www.wildernessmedicinenewsletter.com

For more
information
go to
tmcbooks.com

CPSIA information can be obtained
at www.ICGtesting.com
Printed in the USA
BVOW07s2250230218
508933BV00004B/10/P

9 780982 653920